Grand Mal

D1319857

Grand Mal

A Life with
Late Onset Epilepsy

ROBERT V. DODGE

McFarland & Company, Inc., Publishers
Jefferson, North Carolina

ISBN (print) 978-1-4766-8396-6
ISBN (ebook) 978-1-4766-4166-9

LIBRARY OF CONGRESS AND BRITISH LIBRARY
CATALOGUING DATA ARE AVAILABLE

Library of Congress Control Number 2020047140

Front cover image © 2021 Shutterstock

Printed in the United States of America

*McFarland & Company, Inc., Publishers
Box 611, Jefferson, North Carolina 28640
www.mcfarlandpub.com*

To Larry Dodge,
my brother and hero

Acknowledgments

I would especially like to thank Dr. Danielle McDermott for her assistance in reading this manuscript to check for medical accuracy and her encouragement. I am grateful to McFarland and Managing Editor Susan Kilby for bringing this book to the public. My thanks to Ms. Brittney Thorpe in Johns Hopkins Medical Records for providing my complete records of visits, exams, hospitalizations and operations over the years. I will take this opportunity to express my gratitude to my long-term epilepsy care providers, Drs. Lim Shih Hui and Nei I-Ping in Singapore and Dr. Ronald Lesser in the United States. Most of all, gratitude also goes to my wife Jane who helped me through so much of this and special appreciation to my daughter Anne for her concern. Thanks to my sister Pat and her husband Tom for their hospitality and encouragement throughout. There have been many friends, relatives, and former students who have been supportive, and to all, I express my gratitude for making this situation much more tolerable.

Table of Contents

Preface

About 3.4 million people in the United States and more than 65 million globally suffer from epilepsy and I am one of them. The issues people with epilepsy face are compounded by the difficulties the condition presents to their caregivers, family and friends who exist with the physical hardships and stigma associated with this disorder. Academic books on epilepsy are typically written by doctors who have studied it. The perspective and experience is different for those who actually live with the condition. As an author of academic books who developed epilepsy in my early 30s, I am well aware of what it is like to live with it. Having had seizures and hospital experiences on five continents since developing epilepsy, I have been on 15 different anti-seizure medications and had 15 different neurologists or epileptologists advise me concerning my condition. I've been through four brain surgeries resulting in the removal of one lobe of my brain and several other small sections.

My story is presented to introduce topics in an academic book about epilepsy and to show the reality of a common condition that receives relatively little attention and is widely misunderstood. This has been the case throughout history, both in the West and Asia, as is discussed. That has often led to unfortunate situations for those with epilepsy. The book introduces many subjects basic to understanding epilepsy for both those who have it and those interested in becoming more aware of it. These subjects include the physical aspects of epilepsy and its various forms, including brain structure, seizure types and dangers, pharmaceuticals and side effects, surgeries used to treat it and their various consequences, and the doctor-patient relationship. There are also the social factors associated with the condition, both from society's view and stigmatization as second class citizens, along with the personal view, with frequent depression, driving issues, and employment challenges. While my experiences provide an outline, the discussion is based on extensive research from a wide variety of sources, interviews with those who were with me throughout the time and reports in my medical records.

Introduction

This book begins when I had my first grand mal seizure, an electrical malfunction in my brain that caused me to have violent convulsions. I was 32 and my wife and I were on a camping trip in Morocco. After I returned home and had another seizure, a neurologist diagnosed me as having epilepsy. He placed me on medication and my driver's license was taken for a year. When my National Guard commitment finished, we moved overseas to continue our teaching careers. At the time, epilepsy was commonly associated with mental illness or mental retardation. Explanations of the condition are provided by leading medical authorities. This includes a discussion of whether epilepsy is a disorder or a disease and ramifications of the definitions, along with the economic and legal challenges affecting those disabled by the condition.

Epilepsy involves the brain and seizures. The brain's anatomy and its protection are reviewed, including the hemispheres, lobes, gray matter, dura and more. While the function of each pair of lobes is explained, with the frontal lobe there is brief discussion of surgical prefrontal lobotomy. Seizures are presented as occurring in two broad categories, general and partial, then more specifically defined and classified.

The view that epilepsy and its treatment has involved demons and possession by evil spirits dates back to Neanderthals and the beginning of civilization in Mesopotamia. This continued through the Greeks and Romans, appears in the Bible, was common among Christians of the Middle Ages and has included exorcism for treatment to the present. While demonic possession continued to be believed in the Renaissance, understanding began changing in the 18th century Enlightenment. By the early 19th century there was a search for a natural cause, though many with epilepsy were rejected by society. By the late 19th century the eugenics movement developed and people with epilepsy were considered "defectives." Laws began their incarceration and sterilization as approved by the Supreme Court in the United States, continuing well into the 20th century. In Germany, this was carried farthest under the

T-4 program which involved secret extermination centers for those with epilepsy and others considered "useless eaters" in a precursor to the Holocaust. Restrictive laws continued in the United States to the 1970s.

We moved to England and I faced challenges of stigma or being in denial, trying to hide my condition. The stigma of epilepsy is a burden equal to the physical condition, and many find it the most challenging aspect of having epilepsy. This is a recurring topic, but introductory analysis is based on Ervin Goldman's seminal work plus related topics of felt and enacted stigma, "terrified bystanders," courtesy stigma. We became private school teachers at a school housed in Heywood Manor and received British National Health. Side effects of epilepsy drugs are considered, another recurring topic, as I made drug changes and my dosages of medicine were high. We moved to Singapore where the weather conditions proved to be more challenging for my health. There were new drugs and more seizures. Major life changes also came, including adoption of our child and concern for both her welfare and her attitude about my condition. There was also a sabbatical to Harvard where prescriptions were again changed with little consultation.

Familiarity with the stigma of epilepsy led to my introduction in Singapore to the gold standard of stigmatized people, victims of leprosy. I learned their stories during my 23 years of visiting them weekly and becoming their friend, when their families and the community had abandoned them. They supported me when my circumstances became difficult.

There is in general a low regard in Asia for people with epilepsy. Asian history demonstrates a very long awareness of the condition, but surveys indicate objections to various forms of association with people who have epilepsy. Asian names for the condition provide evidence of attitudes, as they often translate to "madness" or "mad pig disease."

My condition grew worse and my seizures led to hospitalizations. This reached a new extreme when I had an episode of *status epilepticus*, a form of continuous seizure that can be life threatening, and while I managed to get to a hospital, my fate was uncertain. During a relatively long hospitalization I hallucinated much of the time from the drugs needed to halt the seizures and lived in an alternate reality. The experience raised questions on the nature of reality and also convinced me to consider brain surgery. After being released I had more advice on the topic.

When I had a new doctor, a specialist in epilepsy, we discussed epilepsy surgery which he thought was appropriate. Singapore had done the procedure once. I made arrangements to have it done at Johns Hopkins Hospital in Baltimore. The first stage was a stay in the Epilepsy

Monitoring Unit for continuous EEG and video monitoring. Here I nearly died when given a painkiller to which I was allergic. They did the Wada test, which anesthetized each brain hemisphere separately to determine where my speech function was located, and mental testing during my 10-day stay. I found that during partial seizures I was engaging in unusual behavior while thinking I was completely conscious and alert.

After more seizures in Singapore then another in Georgetown requiring hospitalization, I entered Johns Hopkins Hospital for surgery. Friends and family were present, odds had been explained that there was a 70 percent chance of eliminating seizures, a small chance of not surviving the operation, many other possible undesirable results. Seven and a half hours of surgery removed portions of my right temporal lobe, hippocampus, and other small brain structures in the area that seemed to be the origin of seizures. I had difficulties in a 10-day recovery and at one point asked my wife to kill me. It was uplifting to receive get-well greetings from Leprosy Home residents. I improved and was released, but seizures soon followed, and I was shortly back in the monitoring unit. A young girl in the room next to me was recovering from a hemispherectomy, where half of her brain had been removed to prevent very frequent seizures. This operation is discussed as is the adaptability of brain. A severe seizure in the monitoring unit was followed by auditory hallucinations that continued following my release. I went back to Singapore. Dr. Lesser, my doctor from Johns Hopkins, visited and saw the culture and met my Singapore doctor. He explained the next procedure to me that they were going to attempt to eliminate my seizures.

I returned to Johns Hopkins with my wife and daughter. Students sent me 1000 origami paper cranes, many inscribed. This idea came from a famous Japanese book about Hiroshima in the aftermath of the atom bomb. I had a surgery where the flap from previous surgery was reopened plus a hole drilled in the top of my head. Grids with 104 electrodes were placed on the surface of my brain to get an accurate reading of seizure activity. In the monitoring unit following the grid placement, surgery research was conducted on me to do mapping of the brain. They stimulated individual electrodes to record what reactions occurred. This leads to a discussion of the history of locating areas in the brain and corresponding motor function each controlled, dating back to Phineas Gage and efforts to create an accurate homunculus.

The monitoring recorded specific areas where seizures were initiated with secondary spikes elsewhere. Another surgery was then done following a simplistic map from the grid that showed the location of the electrodes, marked ones where the brain beneath it was to be removed.

The operation removed more temporal lobe, also bits of the parietal and occipital lobes. Dr. Lesser said I "have to recognize the fact that I'm handicapped."

I went back to work but had a violent seizure in class in front of my students. My medications were increased well beyond the recommended maximum levels. I was beginning to wonder how I appeared to others, even though I was getting by. When I returned to Johns Hopkins I discussed possibilities and dangers with my doctor who was overseeing my care. He brought up SUDEP (Sudden Unexpected Death in Epilepsy), and this is examined. He also mentioned the possibility of me having a corpus callosum procedure, or severing of the connection between the two hemispheres of my brain, which is also a subject of discussion. I found it disturbing that he would mention this as an option for possibly dealing with my condition. This procedure is used in drastic cases and raises issues beyond medicine, as it can create two individual identities within one head.

I continued to have seizures but had reached the limit of my insurance policy. My school agreed to pay for further surgery and hospitalization. I went back to Johns Hopkins for a fourth surgery. All of the remaining right temporal lobe and the hippocampus were removed, making it about one-eighth of my brain in total.

Following that I had seizures in public places—on a street in downtown Singapore, another on a street in Paris. In both cases people generally ignored me. I had continuous multiple seizures in Aspen that required emergency care. My health was interfering with my daughter's life when I had a seizure outdoors in our neighborhood and she was called on to come to my aid, and another prevented her from getting to her AP exam. Upsetting our loved ones' lives is one of the real regrets for those of us with epilepsy that is considered. There is guilt and shame but no simple alternative. A vagus nerve stimulator was suggested as an option for greater control but I did not proceed to have one implanted.

Instead, I tried new anti-seizure drugs. With one I had an extreme adverse reaction. I encountered a long list of side effects, became near psychotic, was seeing things, could not leave my room for several days. Eventually I had to go through complete medication change in one week, which is considered dangerous and can provoke seizures. Within my first week on a new replacement drug I had status epilepticus after returning from a visit to the leprosy home and was hospitalized in intensive care. The following year I changed medication again, had another status seizure and was in intensive care where survival was questionable. New medicine after that seemed helpful. It was apparent I was no longer stable and my working days were finished. I went on full disability.

We remained in Singapore for a time. While my wife taught, I wrote. I stayed in an isolated cabin over summers where it was dangerous if I had a status seizure again. Once I had incorrect medicine dispensed for my prescription that I used over the summer. Research indicates this is not rare. A new medicine was successful in preventing convulsive seizures, but it was not FDA approved. It was at a time when we were about to return to the United States. At this point, there is a discussion of big pharma and greed. Once the medicine I needed was FDA approved, the same medicine from the same manufacturer at the same dose cost 95 times as much in the United States as in Singapore. There is a similar story from Britain with another drug I used there and continue to use. This is followed by a discussion of generics versus brand name medications for treating epilepsy.

After 35 years as expats we were back in the United States. There is a look at current driving laws and research that indicates people in America with epilepsy are still not welcome and make others feel uncomfortable. There is the condition and the side effects of the medications, and which is affecting one physically and mentally is not always clear. Long standing beliefs in genius paired with insanity have led to many claims of great people in history having had epilepsy which is used to improve the image of the condition. Few of the claims are supported by compelling evidence. Aristotle's observation that people with epilepsy were melancholic is supported by evidence on epilepsy and depression. It is common, as I have felt and found and research supports, for those with epilepsy to feel that they are a burden on others. After 15 medications and four surgeries I still have the condition.

1

Black Blizzards

I was born and raised in Fargo, North Dakota. It was the early summer of 1977, and like nearly all summers since I was in elementary school in the 1950s, I spent much of my time there at Island Park. The park is adjacent to the north-running Red River that separates North Dakota from Minnesota and has over a thousand elm and oak trees of considerable stature, interspersed with pines, on its 35 acres of undulating grassland. My favorite place to be in Island Park was the public tennis courts where I had won five state championships over the years as a doubles player. They had been our home courts for my Fargo Central High and North Dakota State University tennis teams.

In the late summer afternoon at the tennis courts a person was likely to be attacked by swarms of mosquitoes, whether one sat on the wooden benches just outside the chain link fencing that surrounded the concrete courts, or on the park bench under the lean-to roof attached to the "Shack." The Shack was the name given to the one-room wooden hut where I had worked in summers during high school and college, handling court rentals, giving tennis lessons and organizing tournaments. The benches near it were where players would hang around while waiting for a court to be available or relaxing after having played.

While I can never know for certain, it is likely that it was at that favorite place, by the tennis courts, when something unnoticed but important happened. It would have been a late June afternoon, before or after playing tennis, when I was sitting on one of those benches among those swarming mosquitoes that I got one bite that was different; one mosquito out of many that I failed to swat or swish away. This came from an *Aedes* mosquito and it changed my life forever.

My wife, Jane, was visiting her recently widowed mother in California. Jane's father had died tragically young at age 56 of ALS, Lou Gehrig's disease, and her mother was readjusting to the loss and the lifestyle change that accompanied it.

While Jane was away, I began feeling flu symptoms. One evening

I went to a movie but felt dizzy, so I left early and returned home and headed up to our bedroom on the second story of our modest house. When I awoke in the morning my shoulders ached, which seemed strange but not alarming. The soreness continued for days and I told my tennis partners that the flu seemed to have "settled in my shoulders." I visited a walk-in clinic and described my continuing listlessness and fever to a doctor, but neglected mentioning my shoulders, since I had no suspicions and tend to be rather stoic about my health and physical discomfort. That quality would serve me well as things unfolded. He said that as I had suspected it was probably a case of the flu that would soon clear up.

In hindsight, I likely had experienced my first tonic-clonic seizure, formerly known as grand mal, during the night after the movie, and the aching shoulders would be something that would become a more common phenomenon. These seizures are electrical storms in the brain where neurons all fire simultaneously, giving the body directions to do everything at once. This causes convulsions, violent random jerking that is dangerous to the person and his or her brain if they carry on, but they normally stop on their own within a short period.

Unbeknownst to me the mosquito bite I failed to avoid had given me a case of encephalitis, a viral infection that causes inflammation of the brain. Though I recovered quite soon from a presentation of flu-like symptoms of the condition, the disease left residual damage to my brain. That damage was the cause of my epilepsy that emerged that eventful summer and continues to lurk inside me, always waiting to take control.

Jane returned from California and we prepared for a camping vacation in the Atlas Mountains of North Africa. We were both teachers and enjoyed travel, a good combination since we had the work schedules that allowed us to take extended overseas trips, which we had done frequently. Our appetites were whetted for an attempt at international living, but my National Guard commitment had prevented us from considering it seriously until I was discharged, so we went to visit the world—Europe, Tahiti, East Africa, the Amazon and more.

Our flight to the Atlas Mountains included a stopover on the way in London where we went to the theater and sat in the balcony. During intermission, I was walking along holding the railing that dropped to the grand circle and my hearing became jumbled then vanished. I had a strange, slightly disoriented feeling but kept my tingling hand on the railing and tried to make my way through the crowd and find an exit away from the balcony's brink. I recovered so I didn't mention it to my wife. I now know it was an aura, a warning preceding a possible seizure, and something that would become very familiar.

We flew on to Morocco and camping began. After traveling to Casablanca and Marrakesh we set up our tents at a campground outside of Fez and spent several days exploring the fascinating medieval medina, a treat for me as a history teacher. Its narrow streets, often only a meter wide, prevented motorized traffic and were a maze of souks stocked with spices, dates, carpets and various traditional items. Traversing them was perhaps as close as one could come to walking back in time. The most memorable sight was the Leather Souk, the world's oldest leather tannery. The odor was foul but the colors and process spectacular—a honeycomb of stone vessels in sections with many rich colored dying pools, barefoot workers walking on the narrow rims of the vats and using poles to produce fabulous leather products.

While we were seeing the sights of Fez it was extremely hot, upper 90s, and when we returned to our campground of international travelers, Jane changed into a two-piece bathing suit while I went barefoot and put on my swimming suit and a T-shirt. We were preparing to take down our tent to move on. Jane was outside and I entered the tent to pack my things. Jane next heard a loud shout she thought sounded nonhuman. Her immediate thought was that perhaps I'd been shot, but when she entered the tent, she saw me lying on the ground convulsing violently. She grabbed a leather belt of mine and tried to force it in my mouth. That wasn't possible with my jaw clenched, and she screamed for help. Soon others were in the tent, among them our tour guide, and the camp director was contacted.

I stopped convulsing but was incoherent and totally unaware when a flatbed truck arrived and the gathered campers placed me on a stretcher to load me on the back. Jane grabbed clothes since we were in a Muslim country, and with our guide, rode in the cab of the truck to a public hospital. It was a walled facility with security at its entrance. Once we were allowed in, what was found guarded from the public was a very wide circular driveway surrounding a large rectangular structure. At the hospital entrance Jane and others got me off the truck and onto a gurney. She and our guide wheeled me down a hall in search of a doctor. The corridor we followed was dirty and crowded with people attached to IVs, sitting on the floor. The open squat toilets were visible and filthy, as roaches scurried about in the unsanitary conditions.

I was in and out of consciousness by this time and recall soon lying on one of perhaps 20 simple metal frame cots with thin mattresses in a sparsely furnished ward with a concrete floor. This was where the doctors, who all spoke French, saw several patients at once. Jane's French was elementary, while our novice guide's French was only slightly more advanced, so communication was a challenge. Jane tried mimicking a seizure to convey what had occurred and she didn't want me to watch because she was afraid it would trigger another episode. She also didn't want me to know what had happened. I had partially dislocated my shoulder during my convulsions and the doctor made no mention of the seizure, but said she was going to send me down to have someone yank my arm to reposition my shoulder.

At that point, Jane did what would become her habit; she took charge. She is this rather small, trim, dainty person and has always appeared considerably younger than she is, but when my health has been an issue and care was questionable or slow, watch out. She becomes extremely assertive and time after time got me through difficulties I couldn't possibly handle or, in many cases, was not aware that they existed.

She had lost all confidence in this public facility and rather than push the gurney down to the area for shoulder realignment, she and the guide headed to the point where we had entered the building and exited. They managed to get me off the gurney and by this time I could lean against a pillar and remain upright, but no more. It was at least a hundred yards to the entrance of the compound where cars were being let in and the pavement was exceptionally hot. Jane tried chasing the few cars that were admitted to get them to stop, but had no luck. After a time, she and the guide decided they were going to have to get me outside the compound to the main streets where it might be possible to hail a taxi. The guide gave me her flip-flops so I wouldn't burn my feet, as she sacrificed her own. With one arm over Jane and the other over the guide, I was dragged across the hot surface and we made our departure. Outside the hospital compound we secured a ride to our campground.

Upon reaching the campground I was set in the shade of a tree, as it was still extremely hot. With no doctor or medical care, Jane had no idea of what to do next, and I was of no use. It is indicative of her state of mind that one idea she came up with was to buy an airplane to fly to London where we would be safe. She still hadn't told me anything other than I had passed out and hurt my shoulder.

After a while the director of the camp came to say he had found a doctor who could help us. We made arrangements for a driver and went to see him. The doctor was an older French expatriate with a private clinic who had a standup X-ray machine that Jane thought looked like "something out of an old movie." She could see my bones as I stood behind it. The doctor noted my shoulder injury but did not do anything dramatic to realign it. He understood that I had suffered a convulsion and suspected that it was caused by the heat. In his view, it was a febrile seizure rather than epilepsy, so likely a one-off occurrence. This doctor was not a neurologist and he might have meant a "provoked" seizure, as febrile seizures are thought to occur only in children. He prescribed phenobarbital and we returned to the campground to complete our camping trip.

There were six of us who traveled in one van and put all our travel gear in a metal box, which was stored on top when we moved from one location to another. I was the strongest and lifted the box on and off. Following my seizure and as an effect of being on phenobarbital I was groggy and uncertain, so napped in the van frequently and didn't exert myself. The one other man in our group refused to assist with the box and complained about how I had inconvenienced him. The women cooperated and managed to load the box for the remainder of the trip. During that time, Jane told me I'd had a seizure but not how extreme it had been. We weren't too worried, as the doctor had thought it wasn't likely to recur.

Our difficulties weren't over. We made it back to London where we had a direct flight to Winnipeg and when we got on the plane, we sat for seven hours since the Canadian air traffic controllers had gone on strike in early August. My wife cried for the first time as she thought we would never get over "this hellish thing." The flight was diverted to New York then Minneapolis where we boarded buses to Winnipeg. When we returned to the U.S. border and had to stop at customs, Jane found it very difficult to wake me up because the phenobarbital had me sedated.

By the time we returned to Fargo I had an unusual pronounced aura that occurred frequently. Auras are actually focal seizures—seizures that are very localized to one small area of the brain that might excite more neurons and could lead to more visible twitches or even convulsions, but in my case, at that point they just passed away. As my condition later developed, I could feel my aura and gauge whether it was continuing or stopping. If it was continuing it allowed time to prepare for a seizure, so I would be able to find a comfortable spot to get down and not hurt myself.

An unfortunate thing about my aura was that it was brought on by music. This is a trigger for the very unusual, but not unheard of, musicogenic epilepsy. I had been very involved with music—majoring in music in college for a time, paying my college tuition by playing in a dance band and giving music lessons, while being first chair in the university band since my freshman year. I had also spent time in an Army band. Even more, it was near impossible to go through a normal day and avoid music, as it is nearly ubiquitous, on television, in stores, movies, restaurants, elevators, wherever one goes. Being nervous and tentative around music became my way of life. What also became automatic was to be aware of my location and when I stopped, notice the nearest soft spot to get to if my aura persisted so when a seizure came it would cause a minimum of harm.

That failure to swat one mosquito would finish my career as a musician and eventually end my capacity to play tennis as well. Two things I worked hardest at learning to do proficiently would come to exist in reminiscence only, compounding the frustration, as the deterioration of skills took ego along with it. It was a slow process that began with our return to Fargo when a diagnosis emerged.

I made an appointment to see a neurologist at TNI, which stood for The Neuropsychiatric Institute. Dr. Anderson was the doctor I was assigned and he had just finished his residency. He was no older than I and wore cowboy boots as he maintained a very informal, casual manner while we did family history and discussed my medical problems. During our discussion, he concluded from the description of my health during the summer and the outbreak of encephalitis that had occurred in Fargo at that time, that the disease was the likely cause of my difficulties. We next did tests, including flashing lights, and the "skull series" of X-rays, a number of X-rays taken from different angles. On one of the X-rays a dark spot showed up that he couldn't explain. He said he couldn't come to any conclusions, but I watched him add "brain tumor" to his diagnosis pad. Dr. Anderson reduced my phenobarbital and put me on the common anticonvulsant medication Dilantin. He said my seizure remained an anomaly, but if I had a second seizure, state law required him to report it and I would lose my driver's license.

Jane, who had read about seizures and epilepsy since our return, had waited for me. We crossed the street and took a long walk in Island Park, back to where my life's great problem likely began. I told her about the brain tumor diagnosis and we held hands as strolled slowly, discussing things that should be talked about, such as where I would want to be buried, which at age 32 seemed too morbid to consider. That turned out rather premature, but the encephalitis diagnosis would remain the accepted cause.

My older brother came to town to visit the next month and we were all having dinner on the screened-in porch in my parents' backyard. Again, I had an aura brought on by music that generalized to a tonic-clonic, or grand mal seizure. My brother tried to hold me down and my dad attempted to put a spoon in my mouth to keep me from "swallowing my tongue," an impossibility. Jane took command and ordered them to leave me alone while the seizure played out.

I have since heard people, including my doctors in Asia, refer to these occurrences as "fits." While this initially surprised me, I ceased to object, but for anyone who has experienced them, "seizure" is the perfect word for the experience. The feeling is literally that something is coming and then it "seizes you," you completely vanish and are helpless and without defenses in preventing being taken away. This is the sensation, and perhaps because of it, the long tradition of demonic possession that predated neurological understanding came from those with epilepsy as much as those who witnessed their convulsions. More specifically the feeling is your own brain has turned on you and is trying to destroy you. Once a seizure begins you are no longer there, and when it generalizes to what is called complex-partial or especially tonic-clonic and there are convulsions, there is also total amnesia. When I regain consciousness, I have no idea what has transpired or how long it has taken and I'm generally confused for a time, then often tired from an experience I don't know I've had. I'm usually embarrassed, the degree depending on the situation, and always both angry and very disappointed, both for having been victimized by the attack and for again transforming myself into a burden on others. Something came and took "Me" away, which is always frightening.

After the seizure at my parents' house an ambulance came and took me to the hospital where Dr. Anderson had ordered many tests. I had a computerized tomography or CT scan to look for abnormalities in my brain and received an angiogram to check my blood vessels. Following the angiogram I was required to lie on my back to prevent bleeding. It became very uncomfortable and irritating as I wanted to lie on my side, so a group of friends came in intervals to slip their hands behind me and rub my back. They also kept me awake for a sleep-deprived electroencephalogram, or EEG, to measure brain waves and search for any abnormal activity. This test was administered by a former student of mine on the following day. He played the same music, The Eagles, which I had been listening to that brought on my seizure. It worked for getting a spike recorded that indicated a location in my brain that was the likely cause of a problem.

Dr. Anderson also made arrangements for a test that was too late. To see about encephalitis, he ordered a spinal tap. Like the CT scan this also involved someone I apparently knew, but in an awkward reunion. I entered the room for the test and stripped completely, then got on the examination table and assumed the position, which was crouched over resting on my forearms and knees with my face on the table. The high point was my rear end, which was pointed toward the ceiling, and I was completely covered with only my naked butt exposed. A nurse entered who was apparently there to set me at ease and began a conversation. Somehow, she mentioned a name and I said, "I know him." That led in seconds to her saying, "I remember you." It wasn't what I wanted to hear. We had apparently met at some party somewhere and I wasn't going to ask any more about how she remembered me, when all she could see was a high protruding butt surrounded by towels.

Perhaps that succeeded in taking my mind off the spinal tap. It was similar to but more intense than the angiogram, in that the experience wasn't painful. It was just creepy because I could feel something moving inside of me that wasn't supposed to be there.

I was released and my driver's license was taken away. Dr. Anderson increased my Dilantin dosage. Dan, a veterinarian friend, told me he used Dilantin on dogs and could get it for me in bulk at a low price. I took him up on it but my insurance company wasn't willing to accept a statement from a veterinarian clinic, so I went back to a regular pharmacy.

It was time to return to work and things seemed to be going well. I continued to have frequent auras, then one became a convulsive seizure in late November. This was preceded by an aura and happened out of the view of students, but I was taken to the emergency room. Blood work indicated that even though I took the standard dose of Dilantin I wasn't in the "therapeutic range," and I was instructed to increase my daily amount of Dilantin from 300 to 600 milligrams, enough where side effects became a concern. The doctor put me back on phenobarbital as well, and things seemed to improve. Seizures stopped, while auras were reduced. There were minor side effects I was aware of such as slight vision problems. Perhaps there were others that were present in my emotions and facial tics, but none that were obvious to me.

The drug combination seemed to solve my problems for a time and after a year I went in to take my test and get a driver's license again. North Dakota's written exam wasn't much of a challenge at the time. I'd had a driver's license since I was 14 so I had little concern about the driving. When I got in the car with the examining officer, he was rather rude and distant. Not a very "North Dakotan" attitude since it was a small, local highway patrol office. After a time, he asked me why I was taking the exam and everything changed. It seemed apparent he thought I'd lost my license for drunk driving and he wasn't very sympathetic, but when I said I had epilepsy he was fascinated and full of questions about what it was like. The driving finished quickly and I had my license back. In late 1978 I was again driving from Fargo to West Fargo to teach school while Jane continued in Fargo. I continued to have auras but was carrying on a regular life.

There is a strange thing about growing up in North Dakota where you think living in extreme weather is normal. It was the windiest of all states, with Fargo once clocking winds that were forty miles per hour above what qualified as hurricane speed. Temperatures in the state in one year had spanned 181 degrees, from a high of 121° to a low of 60° below zero. Violent thunderstorms might bring hail and destroy a summer's work of farming. Tornadoes, thirteen in the average year, were the most frightening weather events, along with the two or three blizzards that typically struck annually and sometimes unexpectedly. Blizzards could be deadly and they came with "white outs," when visibility was reduced to near zero. Being trapped in the countryside when a storm came up was a real danger. Dying of exposure or freezing could occur in stalled cars or anywhere people were trapped away from shelter. My grandfather had been a variation on this as he drank heavily and regularly in his small town of Mohall and passed out when walking home drunk and was found the next morning dead from exposure, or frozen to death.

In January of 1975 the "Super Bowl Blizzard" crippled neighboring Minnesota, where gale force winds left drifts up to 20 feet deep. In North Dakota only six inches of snow fell on nearly bare ground in what had been a mild winter. There was little snow or ground cover, but the powerful winds mixed dirt from loose topsoil with falling snow into a mixture called "snirt," and there were "snirt storms." For three days, visibility was near zero. Houses were covered with so much snirt that in North Dakota the storm was known as the "Black Blizzard."

Black blizzards had occurred previously in North Dakota and seemed to describe my epilepsy as well as the weather. While blizzards struck and brought white outs, seizures brought blackouts, like black blizzards. With blizzards, there was a real danger that in the wrong conditions they could prove to be deadly. I was to find that seizures were also life threatening, and as time went on that would be the case in the episodes I was having.

Sometimes in the midst of all of this unpleasantness of North Dakota weather you have to tell yourself that nobody is forcing you to stay there. Jane and I had talked at times about living somewhere else and had filled out forms for international school teaching, but never followed up. As with many of our decisions, unseen fortune rather than planning dictated our futures.

Howard Friedberg, the father of one of my students, was active in our school community and I spoke with him frequently. His job was to supervise overseas student teachers for Moorhead State University and he told me that if my wife and I were in Europe when school started, jobs would be available, since teachers didn't show up or became discouraged and had cold feet. When this happened, schools would be desperate to replace them.

My health seemed to be under reasonable control at the time and we were seeking more adventure so we both applied for leaves of absence, which were granted. We were apprehensive about my epilepsy and the stigma attached to it, as it was a common reason for employee discrimination in hiring and retaining workers. That stigma would remain a concern from the time of my diagnosis on, but the choice was to either join in stigmatizing myself by accepting other's prejudices, or ignoring them and seeing how things turned out.

Jane and I rented our house to friends and in the summer, headed to Europe and waited for the school year to begin, hoping that Howard Friedberg was correct. We had no idea at the time, but we were leaving North Dakota permanently and beginning our 35-year lives as expatriates. I was also unaware at the time, that like North Dakota and the changing, extremes and violence of its weather, my own "black blizzards" were with me, buried in my head, waiting to be unleashed in coming years.

2

What Is It?

After being diagnosed as having a seizure disorder, the usual euphemism for epilepsy one first receives, I knew I was an epileptic. That was not the correct word anymore. I had epilepsy. I knew little about it but had vague memories from psychology courses in high school and college of it being discussed in association with mental illness and mental retardation, views that remained commonplace.[1] Doing something about my ignorance would become important, and more so as it became apparent to me that doctors differed considerably in their understanding of the condition.

My prior experience with epilepsy was very limited. When I was in high school, I had seen the older brother of one of my friends have a violent seizure. He was near my locker at Fargo Central High School and when he fell to the floor and began convulsing, I only stood and watched in disbelief. His seizure didn't last long but it was shocking to see him lurching around and twisting, contorting in uncontrolled spasms. Now that's how people would see me, which was disconcerting.

The way my friend's brother approached having epilepsy meant nothing to me at the time, but now I better understand. Though his condition seems to have been under quite good control, he had been a daredevil. He did things that would have been shockingly risky if done by anyone. For a person with epilepsy to have done them, it now seems like he was intentionally tempting fate to a degree where I'm unsure of what he hoped would happen. Depression, low self-esteem, and anxiety commonly accompany epilepsy and I am unaware of whether he felt some sort of mental anguish from having his condition. At that time, such difficulties were not commonly discussed. This is unclear and is a line that I think epilepsy victims frequently tiptoe around, but there are times when we appear to be proving things to others when we're proving things to ourselves.

At the junior high school near us there was a very tall brick smokestack with handrails on one side that extended up about 40 feet. When

I was young, I never dared climb beyond perhaps 10 feet before turning back, but this boy, Curt, who was 13 or 14, climbed to the top. Once he got there, he did a handstand on the chimney's edge that was perhaps six to eight inches wide. He then proceeded to walk on his hands around the rectangular top of the chimney on that narrow edge, after which he returned to his feet and climbed down the hand rails. He did something similar at the stadium where our high school played its football games. By North Dakota standards this was a large arena, a permanent concrete structure rising up on one side of the field with locker rooms underneath. It stood perhaps 25–30 feet with a rail across the back. Curt did an extended handstand on the narrow back rail that dropped off to the ground and a chain-link fence that surrounded the field. A fall in either of these incidents could easily have killed him, and pressure or tension increases the probability of seizures. Falling without a seizure was a very realistic possibility, but for someone with epilepsy this was Russian roulette with extra chambers loaded. Perhaps he didn't care if he fell. I think he was challenging his disease and saying he wasn't going to be its subject or let it define him. It was worth risking his life for him to make those claims.

My other early experience with epilepsy victims was one that I didn't understand at the time. When I was very young, about to turn six, we were on a family road trip to California. We passed a large compound that was fenced in, and running around inside there were many children, some that appeared to be about my age. They were all wearing football helmets. I asked my parents what it was and they gave me some evasive explanation. I realized later it was an institution for epileptics, as being institutionalized for having epilepsy was very common in the United States at that time.

So just what was this thing that I had? According to an article in *Epilepsia*, "Common practice considers epilepsy to be a condition of unprovoked recurring seizures."[2] That seems pretty straightforward. That described my situation and it was how most people understood it. But over the years I would deal with many doctors who would discuss it, offer treatments, change what others had done and mean different things when they used the term "epilepsy." Dr. Anderson had waited until I had my second seizure before reporting me to the drivers' license bureau as a person with epilepsy. He was doing what was a common practice. According to the National Epilepsy Foundation, "A person is diagnosed with epilepsy if they have two unprovoked seizures (or one unprovoked seizure with the likelihood of more) that were not caused by some known and reversible medical condition like alcohol withdrawal or extremely low blood sugar."[3]

It seems pretty clear. Having two seizures meant you have epilepsy. Well, sort of. There's the "unprovoked" and "likelihood" parts that are mentioned. To eliminate confusion, a panel of experts sponsored by the International League against Epilepsy, or ILEA, and the International Bureau for Epilepsy was assigned to make the guidelines for determining specifically what constituted epilepsy. They began by stating, "Little common agreement exists on the definition of the terms seizure and epilepsy," and added, "Such definitions are important for communication among medical professionals as well as with diverse physicians with their patients and their families."[4] Their observation about the importance of precise definition of the vocabulary struck me as very much on point after having had experience with at least 15 different neurologists or epileptologists and being treated for epilepsy by doctors on five continents over the years. I'd found that some doctors speak to their patients and clarify the vocabulary they are using very well, while there are others who speak down to the patient and family as though they couldn't understand. Still others really don't understand so well themselves at times, except to order a blood test, write a prescription.

This panel for ILEA came up with a more precise definition for what constitutes epilepsy. They said a person had it if they experienced at least two unprovoked seizures occurring at greater than 24 hours apart, or one unprovoked seizure and a probability of at least 60 percent of further similar seizures occurring over the next 10 years.[5] The introduction of a specific probability to calculate on whether someone would have a second seizure within 10 years to define that person as having epilepsy made demands on doctors that many were unprepared to meet. While MRIs and scans could lend predictive value about possible problems, unless there were other neurological disorders or deficits evident, this remains very imprecise. A study done following people after having a single seizure found that only about one-third of them had a second when continuing without medication and being unclassified.[6] That's what I'd been hoping after my seizure in Morocco. This uncertainty about accurately knowing whether someone has epilepsy after one seizure raised questions. Should the patient be prescribed medication if he or she will be driving? Should medication be prescribed to someone considering becoming pregnant? The authors of the new ILEA definition of "epilepsy" considered this and said that unless doctors had reason to be able to calculate the specific risk of seizure in an individual situation to diagnose someone as having epilepsy after one seizure, the default position remained two seizures.[7] Another thing about their allowing classification of people as having epilepsy after one seizure caused controversy. There were concerns that this would substantially increase the prevalence of epilepsy.[8] It seems little had changed and I certainly had it.

In recent times, because of the many forms epilepsy can take on, the ILEA experts noted that "epilepsy is not one condition, but is a diverse family of disorders, having in common an abnormally increased predisposition to seizures. Some writers prefer the plural term, 'the epilepsies.'"[9] That this usage is becoming accepted is seen in the National Institute of Health's story on seizures, "The Epilepsies and Seizures: Hope Through Research."[10] I will certainly pass on it even though my condition has taken a number of forms. Just one epilepsy is plenty.

What appears to have provided more division is determining epilepsy's classification. MedicineNet treats "epilepsy" and "seizure disorder" as synonyms, interchangeable names.[11] The Epilepsy Foundation describes it as a "chronic disorder."[12] The World Health Organization's phrase for epilepsy is "noncommunicable disease of the brain."[13] Recognized U.S. authorities Jerome Engel, Jr., and Timothy A. Pedley say, "Epilepsy is not a specific disease, but a broad category of symptom complexes arising from a variety of disordered brain functions."[14] The Mayo Clinic defines it as a "central nervous system (neurological) disorder."[15] Some advocates believe that referring to epilepsy as a "disorder" or something not well understood by the public minimizes the seriousness of the serious nature of the condition. Major international epilepsy advocacy organizations recommended in 2014 that it is best that epilepsy be considered to be a disease.[16]

Whether epilepsy is a disorder or a disease may seem like an insignificant point. It seems not unlikely that among those who would prefer the distinction would be advocacy groups who believe disease might make epilepsy seem a more serious condition to the public so they could more easily raise awareness, and I would assume funds. If you have a disease, you're sick. Mackelprang and Salsgiver point out what this means in Western society: "People with disabilities, whom society assumes are 'sick,' are expected to fill this role even when they are perfectly healthy. Their only obligation is to be grateful for the help given them, thus subjecting them to a form of benevolent oppression."[17] "Benevolent oppression"—this is often a result of good intentions, where people who are caretakers do not trust the person with epilepsy to be able to make good decisions or handle problems on his or her own, yet that person wants to feel normal and like everyone else and to be seen that way by the people he or she meets in school or other social situations. Unfortunately, the evidence is that epilepsy tends to lead to feelings of isolation and is a barrier to feeling "normal"[18] to many people.

The issue of describing epilepsy a disorder or a disease hints at a major approach-avoidance conflict in how it is defined. As with other stigmatized conditions, this affects all concerned: those with it and the life they will lead, their families and friends, their care providers, their employers, the government. It is very important for people with epilepsy to be seen as "normal" and like everyone else in many situations, such as when they apply for jobs. Then there's the other side, where if they are normal, do they need legal protection against discrimination? Who will protect them if their employer finds out they have epilepsy and decides to let them go and not take any chance something bad will happen, even though they are doing fine at their job? Threading this needle of being normal enough to hold jobs and be accepted while being legally protected against discrimination because of a disability has been the challenge.

Prejudice against people with handicaps has a long tradition. It was sanctioned by the Bible in both the Old and New Testaments.[19] In earlier times it had been assumed that problems people with disabilities faced, including finding work or getting an education, were the inevitable consequences imposed upon them by their physical or mental disability and how their lives should be.[20] Even during much of the 20th century people with disabilities such as epilepsy were long not included as a legally protected class. The civil rights movement led to the Civil Rights Act of 1964[21] which prohibited private sector discrimination in employment against women, racial and ethnic minorities, and banned discrimination against minorities in public accommodations. Protections for the handicapped were not included.

It was in 1973 with the passage of Section 504 of the 1973 Rehabilitation Act that for the first time, the exclusion and segregation of people with disabilities was viewed as discrimination. Section 504 stated: "No otherwise qualified handicapped individual ... shall, solely by reason of his handicap, be excluded from the participation in, be denied the benefits of, or be subjected to discrimination under any program or Federal activity receiving Federal assistance."[22]

Court battles and more organized advocacy followed. Various groups representing people with different handicaps combined to put pressure on congress for meaningful legislation. In 1985, 14 percent of the U.S. population that was not institutionalized reported having a disability that limited their ability to function.[23] The average income for disabled men was $18,423 compared with $30,376 for those without disabilities.[24] A comprehensive study concerning epilepsy in the mid–1980s found that "people with epilepsy at all levels of severity are significantly less likely to work than people without the disorder" and not surprisingly, those whose seizures were more severe were significantly less likely to work than those whose seizures were less impairing.[25] Simply having epilepsy reduced wages by approximately $2.50 per hour.[26] They found epilepsy was a greater employment deterrent for men than for women, though this called for more analysis.[27]

Having epilepsy clearly put people at a disadvantage, even when their disorder did not interfere with their capability to work productively and successfully. Legal equality could benefit them and there were very active groups working to achieve it, coupling their efforts with similar organizations that represented people who suffered from other conditions. What those with epilepsy and other disabilities had hoped for in terms of legal protection came on July 26, 1990. In front of 3000 people assembled on the White House lawn President George H.W. Bush stated, "This historic act is the world's first comprehensive declaration of equality for people with disabilities—the first,"[28] as he signed into law the Americans with Disabilities Act,[29] commonly referred to as the ADA. This law banned discrimination on the basis of disability in employment, public housing and services, transportation, telecommunications. Regulations for employment provisions and the Equal Employment Opportunity Commission were soon added.

I was away for this but aware it was happening. As for my own definition, whether it's a sickness or a disorder is of little importance. I had seizures and they weren't all the same. That meant I had epilepsy.

3

What Happens

There are many kinds of epilepsy experiences. Two things that are constant are that they always involve seizures and those always originate in the brain. The three-pound squishy mass of fat and protein that makes up the brain is not only the most complex structure in the body. With 100 billion neurons making more than 100 trillion interconnections,[1] it has been described as the most complex thing in the universe.[2] Damage to the brain can cause seizures as in the case of my encephalitis, or as a result of head injuries or brain tumors among other things. The brain has considerable protection in many ways.

The brain is guarded from damage in all but the most extreme assaults from the outside by being encased in a very hard covering of bone, the skull. Below the skull there is the dura, an inflexible membrane with an outer layer for protection and an inner layer that lines all the skull and has folds that create compartments or divisions for protection and separating parts of the brain. Another layer of elastic tissue is below the dura that carries blood vessels. One more layer of tissue lies below that covers the surface of the brain and allows for the flow of cerebrospinal fluid. Cerebrospinal fluid is a clear, watery substance that not only flows around the brain but also fills cavities in the brain called ventricles.

With this protection from blunt force trauma and cushioning, many problems can be halted, but the brain's protection does not stop there. Of special importance is the blood-brain barrier. This is a semi-permeable membrane that gives special protection to the brain by acting as a gatekeeper on the blood that enters the organ. It admits the necessary blood to provide nutrients and oxygen but prevents harmful substances including poisons and some disease-causing viruses from entering. While it is not perfect, it prevents many things that manage to enter the body from reaching the brain where they could cause great problems. At a more reduced level, the brain consists of neurons and glial cells. There are types of glial cells that provide physical protection to neurons and help keep them healthy. In another show of the brain's adaptability in protecting itself researchers have found that it appears to develop its own immune system on a short-term basis. The body's regular immune system doesn't pass the blood-brain barrier as it might wreak havoc on neurological functions. What was discovered was that to protect itself, a specific, limited immune response develops to certain unwanted assaults on the brain, then it disappears before causing other problems.[3]

The structure of the brain is categorized and subdivided.[4] It is common to begin with three main components, the brainstem, the cerebellum and the cerebrum. The brainstem is the most primitive part and is connected to the spinal cord. Among its functions are to control breathing, blood pressure, and heart rhythms and it is the message center between the body and the thinking parts of the brain. Damage to this can cause "brain death." In the very back of the head is the cerebellum. It is separated by a fold of dura. This area is associated with fine motor movements of the fingers and also posture, balance, control of the limbs.

The major part is the cerebrum that is 85 percent of the brain's weight, and often thought of as the brain. It has an outer surface called the cerebral cortex with billions of neurons that is very wrinkled and is called the "gray matter" due to its color. Because of the vast number of elaborate convolutions in this layer which is only an eighth of an inch thick,[5] it has a surface area of 310 square feet,[6] allowing for the advanced functioning of the human mind. It is thought that it is this layer that distinguishes the human brain from that of other animals.[7] Below this is the main structure of the cerebrum which is made of white matter. The cerebrum has two parts, a right and left hemisphere, that are joined by a cable of nerves known as the corpus callosum, where messages are delivered from one half to the other. One side is usually functionally dominant and controls speech and language, though there are cases where this dominance is mixed. The left side of the brain controls movement on the right side of the body and vice versa. In the cerebrum, there are fissures that separate area into regions called lobes.

The lobes come in pairs with one on each hemisphere. The largest are the frontal lobes, sitting behind the forehead. These lobes are involved in thinking, learning, movement, emotions, judgment, problem solving. The importance of these lobes has made surgery on them controversial. After World War II there was common use of prefrontal lobotomy to treat patients suffering from severe depression or schizophrenia and 50,000 were carried out in the United States between 1942 and 1954.[8] The side effects sometimes included emotional and mental distress and personality changes to the point of people being reduced to what were sometimes classified as "vegetative states."[9] John

Kennedy's sister Rose was one of the early subjects of the operation when her father was told it would improve her irritability and backwardness,[10] and the public knows of it from the book and movie *One Flew Over the Cuckoo's Nest*.[11] The practice was revived somewhat in the 1960s and '70s but has since been challenged on the basis of the inability of patients to give informed consent. The time eventually came when I had discussions with my doctor about having surgery to remove something in my frontal lobe, but because there seemed to be much too much at stake in terms of major problems, I never gave it serious consideration.

As for other lobes, in the back of the brain are the occipital lobes. These deal with visual information, process colors and give meaning to shapes. The parietal lobes receive information from other areas to manage body position and sensation. On the side of the brain about ear level are the temporal lobes. These are involved in memory and hearing and help with recognition of faces as well as understanding language. A section of them also is involved in interpreting other people's emotions and reactions. In all, this makes four pairs, so eight lobes. A temporal lobe would become my major problem and concern, though all lobes on one side would eventually either have surgical intervention or be considered for it.

While the brain is phenomenally complex and well protected, there are times for some people when the connections called synapses malfunction and can lead to abnormal electrical activity. This can lead to seizures. It is most common for this to happen in babies under the age of one or seniors over 65, when other brain problems such as strokes, Alzheimer's disease, and tumors are more common problems and may cause seizures.[12] Traumatic injury and certain illnesses can lead to seizures. They can take on many different forms, affect different people in different ways, and are sometimes referred to as "electrical storms" in the brain.[13] That phrase is similar to the classic definition of an epileptic seizure provided by Hughlings Jackson in 1870 as "an occasional and a disorderly discharge of nerve tissue."[14]

The Epilepsy Foundation's description of what happens during a seizure mentions that some people experience a "prodrome," which is not actually part of the seizure, but a warning that can occur even days before that it is coming.[15] I went through a period before having surgery when I would think I had "auras of auras." These were just slight unusual feelings, somewhat more like panic than something in my head, that I was going to have an aura sometime in the next week. It seems in recollection that I found them to be quite accurate, but having auras was also common, so there may not have been a correlation. A recent study has described similar occurrences, but not determined their accuracy in predicting auras or seizures to follow.[16] Some people have an aura, or warning, and I was fortunate to be one of them. Mine could just be a tingling in my left hand, or the hearing loss I mentioned. They could take many forms. For some this is a strange taste or odor, a feeling in the stomach, sudden joy or sorrow, a feeling like a "wave" going through the head. Others report more psychic experiences, such as flashing lights, hallucinations, a feeling of déjà vu, the sensation a leg or arm has changed in size.

Accompanying auras, some common effects are feelings of fear or panic, racing thoughts, racing heart, dizziness or lightheadedness, numbness or tingling, blurry vision. As the seizure spreads, more outward symptoms will become visible, such as minor shaking, fumbling, chewing, possibly muscle stiffening. The aura is in the category of focal seizure, and you are completely conscious, but is considered the beginning of a seizure. By the time the symptoms begin to assert themselves, you are aware that something is happening beyond your aura, though the degree of awareness determines the classification of the seizure. If it doesn't progress and remains in one sensory or motor area of the brain, and the person remains awake and understands what is happening, it is called a simple partial seizure or focal onset aware. If the person is confused and their awareness is affected, it is a complex partial, or focal impaired. Once the seizure has begun it has entered what is known as the ictal phase.

Over 40 types of seizures and many more syndromes have been identified.[17] Only a small number are widely known and diagnosed. Seizures are commonly divided into two categories, generalized or partial, sometimes called focal, depending on how and where they begin in the brain. When there was no witness or way of determining the beginning of the seizure it would be classified as "unknown onset."

In the generalized seizure category, there is the tonic-clonic seizure that was known previously by the name "grand mal." The onset of these seizures can be generalized but they can evolve from focal seizures if the seizures continue to spread until they take over both halves of the brain. Another word for this is convulsion, and some people use fit, which I would find was common in some places outside the United States. Perhaps that is acceptable since they have different traditions of cultural usage and phrases, but it seems unacceptable in America. Expressions of insult here include fit to describe outrage ("When my parents saw my grades they threw a fit") or tantrum ("She had a hissy fit when they didn't have the dress in her size"). Since those are insulting references to an experience of people with epilepsy, the use of the word is then an insult to the people who have the condition as well and an improper choice, also something best avoided when in the company of people with epilepsy. Tonic-clonic seizures are what most people commonly think about of as seizures and are stereotyped as foaming at the mouth, biting the tongue. The name combines two types of seizures that are phases of this event. First is the "tonic" phase when muscles stiffen and the person will suddenly lose consciousness, so will fall to the ground if caught unaware. The muscles are stiff and the air is forced out, which can cause it to sound like a scream or cry, known as the "ictal cry" and what my wife heard in Tunisia that caused her to come to our tent. The tonic phase is brief, lasting only seconds, then the clonic phase begins which is the part that involves convulsions. This carries on sometimes only for seconds but often for a minute or two. It is a good idea to time it, if you happen to be present for this phase. If it continues for over five minutes from the seizure onset, contact 911 or seek emergency help. The same is true if it stops, then starts up again and repeats that another time, as multiple seizures also demand emergency care. This can be a condition called status epilepticus, when the seizure just continues and doesn't stop on its own, creating considerable risk to the person as I would eventually discover.

Absence, or petit mal, seizures are another type of generalized seizures that affect both hemispheres. They rarely start before the age of two or after the teenage years. These are brief seizures, sometimes only a few to 30 seconds, where mental functioning abruptly stops, responsiveness is absent, memory is not functioning. There may be facial changes, most frequently blinking, or the person remains motionless and stares. Some movements, called automatisms, might take place, possibly grimacing, chewing, fumbling with clothes. The person receives no aura or warning and is not fatigued by the event, so may not be aware it took place unless there is a clue of lost time.[18]

Other generalized seizures include myoclonic seizures are typically jerks and can be very large contractions of the limbs, head and thorax. They often look like clumsiness or having gotten up on a foot that was asleep. This involves rapid, brief contractions of muscles that occur on both sides of the body at the same time, though they might involve only one foot or arm. Dravet syndrome is a severe myoclonic epilepsy of infancy, with a presentation of multiple seizure types. It falls in a category of epileptic encephalopathy in infants where seizures are multi-form, cognitive, behavioral and neurological deficits are possible, and early death is a danger. Also in this category is the rare Lennox-Gastaut syndrome in children, which was found to be nearly immune to treatment and has caused learning problems. There was pressure on behalf of victims of Dravet syndrome and Lennox-Gastaut syndrome to make an unprecedented change in legal treatment allowed to these poor victims whose families were desperate for what was thought to be a helpful treatment. In 2018, the Federal Drug Administration approved the use of a CBD medicine, derived from cannabis, for children two years and older. This was after three randomized, double-blind, placebo-controlled clinical trials found what some of the parents already knew. Use of CBD from cannabis was effective in reducing seizures when compared with a placebo.[19]

Another kind of seizures that are usually general and can be dangerous are atonic seizures, also known as "drop seizures" or "drop attacks." Though these are usually very brief, lasting only seconds, the name means "without tone" and that describes them. The body suddenly goes limp and if the person is standing or walking, he or she falls. If sitting, the person slumps over. Unlike a tonic-clonic seizure there is no long recovery time where the person is groggy and confused, but there is considerable risk of injury or disaster depending on the circumstances. A study of a substantial number of people with the condition found "epileptic drop attacks are extremely disabling, both because of the continuous traumatic risk and for the need for patients to be accompanied or move only in a wheelchair or when wearing a helmet."[20] This study also concluded that these debilitating seizures were "characteristic of patients with Lennox-Gastaut syndrome,"[21] adding to the complications these children face.

The number of people in the United States who endure some form of seizure is 3.4 million and the number of children is approaching a half million.[22] With some like me it is an infrequent experience and with others, they strike hundreds of times a day as the protection system built for our precious brains lets us down. There are antiepileptic drugs for this and it is estimated that in America 50 percent of people with epilepsy will gain complete control over their epilepsy for substantial periods of time by taking their medications, while another 20 percent will see a significant reduction in seizures. There are others for whom medication does not supply a solution for their problem. They are often described as having intractable epilepsy, which was my eventual diagnosis. For these people, they can wait and hope some new drug will be developed or that things in some different combination might be an improvement and there sometimes can be other options.

4

Demons

I was beginning to survive with relatively few difficulties by taking daily medication. It was the late 1970s, and at that point, my awareness was that having epilepsy meant I was mentally ill or mentally retarded and that people with epilepsy could be institutionalized or so threatened by their condition that they would do anything to overcome it and the horror of living with it. In contrast to this, I was feeling quite normal. So as a history teacher I did what seemed reasonable—looked to the past to see where the attitudes about epilepsy had originated and how widespread they were. This was something I have continued as my condition went through many changes and it has consistently been an unpleasant story.

There is evidence that the first use of à surgical instrument for an incision was intended to alleviate epilepsy and dates back to long before civilization.[1] This was trepanning, the cutting or drilling of a hole in the skull of a human. This practice began with Neanderthal Man and it is thought that for much of its early history the purpose was to allow an escape point for the evil spirit that was possessing the victim. Surprisingly, this practice was the only form of brain surgery available for epilepsy for many thousands of years, and it continued to be used from these early forms of man around the world as they emerged until the end of the 1700s, with different justifications along the way.[2] The 19th century would bring new experiments, and modern epilepsy surgery began in 1886 in London, 110 years before I had the first of my experiences with it.

Written reports of epilepsy date back to about 2000 BC. The first mention of the condition comes from Akkadia in Mesopotamia with a description of a person who foamed at the mouth while his neck turned left and his hands and feet were tense, his eyes wide open until he lost consciousness. The diagnosis of this condition was as *antašabbû*, which meant the victim was under "the hand of Sin," the god of the moon and father of the sun.[3] In ancient cultures it was standard to regard disease as supernatural, a punishment or curse from the gods or evil spirits, or reprisal for sins.[4] This associating of epilepsy and having seizures as retribution for sin would remain throughout antiquity and the Middle Ages,[5] while it being a result of religious or demonic possession would be an enduring theme that continues to contemporary times.

A case that received some attention about the time I developed epilepsy was that of Anneliese Michel, a 22-year-old German student who was anorexic and suffered from frequent seizures. Her parents contacted their local parish priest who considered the seizures to be an indication of possession rather than epilepsy, and he consulted with Germany's leading "satanologist" who confirmed this. The parish priest called in an expert and for ten months they conducted exorcisms to drive out the devils, thought to number at least six, and calling themselves among other things Lucifer, Judas, Nero, Hitler.[6] Throughout the time, Anneliese ate and drank almost nothing and grew progressively weaker to a point of severe malnutrition. During a violent session, she rushed a wall and smashed her head, then collapsed back on her bed. With that, the priests declared the devils had left her, and in the morning, she was found dead. In 1978, two years later, the two priests and Anneliese Michel's parents were tried and found guilty of negligent homicide for not seeking medical attention for the girl.[7] Two decades later, when I was about to have my fourth brain surgery, another report of possession ending in tragedy came from Egypt, stating, "Police detained an exorcist after a woman with epilepsy was beaten to death with a stick and belt, allegedly in an attempt to rid her of four spirits believed to be causing her seizures."[8] More recently, a survey found that a substantial proportion of Saudi Arabians of both genders and of all education levels believe in *Jinn* demonic possession as a cause of epilepsy.[9]

The Code of Hammurabi in ancient Babylon that dates from 1780 BC is often cited as outlawing marriage to epileptics[10] in an early form of eugenics. It included a provision that would allow a man who unknowingly married a woman with a "latent defect" such as epilepsy to divorce her,[11] and a slave sold with epilepsy could be returned for full price.[12] Egyptian surgical papyruses from about the same time indicate an awareness of epilepsy that describes patients with convulsions who "shudder exceedingly."[13]

The Babylonian medical text known as *Sakikku*, or "All diseases," that dates back to the 11th century BC contains the earliest detailed description and explanation of epilepsy and can still be viewed at the British Museum in London. It includes two clay tablets that were devoted entirely to *antašubba* and *miqtu*, which in the Sumerian and Akkadian languages of the time translate as "the falling disease."[14] This became a common name for epilepsy from that point on. These writings go into surprising detail about auras and different forms of seizures, and identify various demons or ghosts responsible for each. Armed with this information, the medical practitioner or exorcist of the time, known as the *āšipu*, could determine how to confront the demon he was facing. Frequently this would be *Lilû* or his wives *Lilītu* and *ardat Lilî*, but among others causing specific seizure activity were *sibit etemni*, the *e'ē-lu*-demon, an encircling *bennu*-demon and "seizure by ghosts."[15] An *āšipu* from 3000 years ago who was familiar with the *Sakikku* would have been more likely to have diagnosed me correctly than the first doctors I encountered in Morocco, as the first thing my wife noticed was my inhuman shout. The ancient text notes, "If he cries '*u āyi!*' or utters a sound like an animal ... it is *miqtu* (epilepsy)."[16]

This artifact includes the first references to what would become my greatest challenge, status epilepticus, or status seizures, those that don't stop or continue to recur. Two references accurately note the seriousness of these as I would find out: "If an epilepsy demon falls many times upon him on a given day he seven times pursues and possesses him, his life will be spared. If he should fall upon him eight times his life may not be spared," and "If an epilepsy demon falls upon him many times and on a given day he seven times pursues him and he has a fit with a loss of consciousness.... He will die."[17]

Greek civilization brought a change in awareness but still considerable misunderstanding. The name "epilepsy" is originally derived from the Greek verb *epilambanein*, which means "to seize, possess." In early times the condition was considered divine punishment and was associated with having offended Selene, the Goddess of the Moon.[18] Galen of Pergamon, who would be the leading medical authority of ancient times, contended that the phases of the moon governed cases of epilepsy.[19] This association of epilepsy with the moon and its phases gave it another enduring name. The Roman equivalent for Selene was Luna, their Goddess of the Moon. People with epilepsy were moonstruck or "lunatics," which would also become associated with mental illness. While some made a distinction between those possessed by gods ("lunatics") and those possessed by demons ("maniacs"), the lunatic label would continue to be applied to people with epilepsy and they would be confined as mentally ill into the 20th century.[20] A belief the Greeks held that would echo through the ages was that epilepsy was a contagious condition.

Aristotle declared that because of a surplus of black bile, those with epilepsy tended to be "melancholic."[21] As was so often true, he was a great observer. A recent study found that people with epilepsy are at least twice as likely to suffer from depression as those who do not have it.[22] Aristotle also wrote that seizures were a form of sleep, and suggested prophetic vision might occur during the experience.[23] This would lead later Romans, Neo-Platonic philosophers and eventually Thomas Aquinas in the Middle Ages to adopt the view of some with epilepsy as shamans or prophets. The name *divinatio* was suggested by some as a synonym for epilepsy.[24] While stigma and persecution has been the story of those with epilepsy, the notion that some are possessed with divine vision has persisted throughout history and some of the most influential individuals, including among others Buddha, St. Paul and Joan of Arc, suffered from the condition.[25]

The Father of Medicine, Hippocrates, is given credit for challenging the view of epilepsy being a result of possession with his *On the Sacred Disease*,[26] written about 400 BC. Epilepsy was known as the sacred disease because it came from Selene and certain features of seizures were attributed to other gods, including Apollo, Poseidon, Hermes.[27] He rejected the idea that epilepsy had a religious or spiritual cause and contended it was a natural illness. This was made clear in his first sentence: "It is thus with regard to the disease called Sacred: it appears to me to be nowise more divine or more sacred than other diseases, but has a natural cause from which the originates like other affections."[28] Another lasting observation he made was where this disorder is located. He wrote, "The brain is the cause of this affection, as it is of other great diseases, and in what manner and from what cause it is formed, I will now plainly declare."[29] As with Greeks of the time he believed health was a balance of humors, phlegm, and bile and their effects on air and blood, along with external factors such as wind and moisture. An imbalance was responsible for epilepsy. The name he gave to the condition was "great disease" which in Latin would become "mobus maior." When it reached Medieval France it became "grand mal," a name that lasted to the present as a designation for a major epileptic seizure.[30]

Hippocrates also was aware of auras and the stigma of having epilepsy. He wrote, "Persons as are habituated to the disease know beforehand when they are about to be seized and flee from men; if their own house be at hand, they run home, but if not, to a deserted place, where as few as possible will see them falling, and they immediately cover themselves up. They do this from shame of the affection, and not from fear of divinity, as many suppose."[31] How little things have changed in 2,400 years. Hippocrates' great work presented the idea that epilepsy is inherited when he stated, "What is to hinder it from happening that where the father and mother were subject of this disease, certain of their offspring should be so affected also"[32] This would remain a controversy in the study of epilepsy from that point on. He also claimed that people are born with the condition, writing, "It begins to be formed while the fetus is still in utero."

This belief that epilepsy was a condition one was born with had consequences. There is evidence that newborn babies with epilepsy in the ancient Greek warrior city-state of Sparta were "exposed." After their birth, all males were given an initial inspection by city elders that involved submersion in wine or urine that was thought to induce seizures in those born with epilepsy. Those who reacted were placed alone in the countryside and left to starve, die of thirst or be prey for animals.[33]

In Ancient Rome, it apparently was not a similar deterrent to success, at least among the patrician, or upper class. One name given to epilepsy was *comitialis morbus* because if a senator of assemblyman had a seizure during the assembly (*comita*) the session had to be canceled.[34] For common people having epilepsy was a considerable problem, as it was considered contagious and spitting on those who were suffering from it was standard practice. This was to repel the cause of the disease.[35] Treatment remained the great problem, as many still believed in possession, and effective medications failed to produce results. Among the cures that didn't involve magic, Galen prescribed drinking burnt human bones.[36] Physicians' prescriptions indicate both their lack of any idea of what might be useful and how desperate those with the condition were, as they were willing to try anything. Medications included hippopotamus and boar testicles, seal and hare genitals, tortoise blood, camel's hair, poultry and ram cock, a medicine composed of the blood of a sea tortoise, the genitals and heart of a hare and the feces of the land crocodile.[37] In folk medicine there were amulets, chants, purging, enemas, shaving the head as well as less expensive medicines, including among them rain water from a human skull, the fat and blood of a black dog, and crushed flea swallowed in egg.[38] The cure that some claimed to have found effective was the warm blood of slain gladiators.[39] This was described by Pliny:

> Epileptic patients are in the habit of drinking the blood even of gladiators, draughts teeming with life, as it were; a thing that, when we see it done by the wild beasts even, upon the same arena, inspires us with horror at the spectacle! And yet these persons, forsooth, consider it a most effectual cure for their disease, to quaff the warm, breathing, blood from the man himself, and, as they apply their mouth to the wound, to draw forth his very life; and this, though it is regarded as an act of impiety to apply the human lips to the wound of even a wild beast! Others there are, again, who would make the marrow of the leg-bones, and the brains of the infants, the objects of their research![40]

While remedies were hopeless and the commoners were still generally seen as possessed, it was a victim of epilepsy who achieved the greatest power and fame, Julius Caesar. His bouts with seizures are well recorded by scholars from the early Roman Empire and also made famous by Shakespeare, but they did not interfere with his military and political genius. His epilepsy was unusual in that it was late onset, not afflicting him until he was age 54.[41] Plutarch wrote that Caesar was "subject to an epilepsy," which, it is said, "first seized him at Corduba."[42] He also suggests there was an aura that preceded Caesar's seizures: "He was too far disordered his senses, when he was already beginning to shake under its influence, withdrew into neighboring fort where he reposed himself."[43] The belief that Caesar had epilepsy has been questioned recently since a letter to a journal suggested that his symptoms could be explained as the result of a stroke.[44] While this view received some attention in the press[45] it was not the subject of historical or neurological journals from that time after, so it appears the academic community has remained convinced by the epilepsy diagnosis.

Shortly after Caesar's rule Christianity was born. This was not a step forward for epilepsy care since where Hippocrates had looked for natural causes, this marked a return to possession by an evil spirit as the reason for the condition. Epilepsy is described in the Bible in Mark 9: 14–29 in a story of an encounter involving a boy who suffered from seizures who met Jesus. The boy's father begins the story, "Master, I have brought unto thee my son, which hath a dumb spirit; And wheresoever he taketh him, he teareth him: and he foameth, and gnasheth with his teeth, and pineth away … and when he saw him, straightway the spirit tare him; and he fell on the ground, and wallowed foaming."[46]

From this description, it appears the boy suffered from tonic-clonic seizures. Upon seeing this, "Jesus … rebuked the foul spirit, saying unto him, 'Thou dumb and deaf spirit, I charge thee, come out of him, and enter no more into him.' And the spirit cried, and rent him sore, and came out of him." As for the boy, "he was as one dead; insomuch that many said, He is dead. But Jesus took him by the hand, and lifted him up; and he arose."[47] This also sounds tonic-clonic, as it is common to fall into deep sleep immediately following the seizure. The passage created the belief that was shared by many priests, both in the Roman and Orthodox churches, that epilepsy was caused by an "unclean dumb and deaf spirit," and those with epilepsy were "demoniacs."[48]

Christianity, which was the Catholic Church of Rome, dominated the Middle Ages. The Catholic belief in the "dark ages" following the fall of the Roman Empire was that persons with epilepsy were possessed by demons and other evil forces. The Catholic Church remained officially unfriendly to those with epilepsy into the current times. Men with epilepsy were banned from attending Catholic seminaries until 1983.[49] As far as marriage to patients with epilepsy is concerned, the Catholic Church's law, canon law, continues to state that epilepsy may interfere with capacity for marital consent and therefore, render marriage to a person with epilepsy invalid from the start, annulling the marriage.[50] Because the condition was considered to be contagious, it was common to segregate those who had it, out of fear that they would contaminate the communion plate and cup.[51] Since early man, exorcism to drive out evil spirits and demons has been a tool for dealing with epilepsy victims and the Catholic Church formalized this into a religious rite. While the practice is not frequent, it continues, as is related in the book *An Exorcist Tells His Story*.[52] Father Amorth relates the story of a sainted exorcist, Father Candido, who performed an exorcism on a patient who had been treated by a psychologist:

> Father Candido was exorcising a young man who was diagnosed with epilepsy by the psychiatrist who was advising him. The doctor accepted the invitation to watch his young patient during an exorcism. When Father Candido touched the head of the youth with his hand, he fell to the ground in convulsions. "You see, Father, that we are obviously dealing with epilepsy," the doctor quickly pointed out. Father Candido bent down and again put his hand on the youth's head. He jumped up and remained motionless. "Is this what epileptics do?" asked Father Candido. "No, never," answered the psychiatrist, obviously taken aback by that behavior. Father Candido's exorcisms eventually completely cured the young man, while for years, doctors and prescriptions—not to mention the high fees—had only harmed him.[53]

While driving out the demons was the accepted method for dealing with those with epilepsy, for a time things took a turn for the worse for many in the late Middle Ages. In response to heresies the Catholic Church adopted a new strategy called the inquisition. This Catholic inquiry by a friar who both judged and handed out sentences led to 32,000 executions in Spain alone, largely of Muslims and Jews.[54] It was in this context that Pope Innocent VIII issued the papal bull, or edict, *Summis Desiderantes* in 1484, directing Dominicans Johann Sprenger and Heinrich Kraemer to prepare a work to stop the advance of witchcraft. The document they produced would become the standard guidebook on witchcraft for the next two centuries not only for Catholics but also for Protestants who emerged soon after its production in the late 1480s.[55] This also coincided with the new printing press, making its availability vastly more widespread. Their work titled *Malleus Malleficarum* (the Witch's Hammer) was based on Exodus 12:18, "Thou shalt not suffer a witch to live." Thus began a witch hunting craze that was endorsed by the Pope as well as the leaders of the new Protestant religions, Martin

Luther and John Calvin.[56] Although no records were kept, it is estimated that between the early 14th century and 1650 between 200,000 and 500,000 people were executed in continental Europe as witches and 85 percent or more were women.[57]

The guidebook for this, *Malleus Malleficarum,* makes reference to epilepsy, but in what seems an odd consistency for me because of later experiences, the mentions are paired with leprosy. This is how epilepsy is presented: "Witches are able to cause leprosy or epilepsy"[58]; "Remedies which can be applied in the case of those infirmities which we have been discussing are equally applicable to all other infirmities, such as epilepsy or leprosy"[59]; "But there is no bodily infirmity, not even leprosy or epilepsy, which cannot be caused by witches, with God's permission."[60]

Women with epilepsy were singled out and targeted in the near mass hysteria where the unusual and weak in the population were victimized as witches.[61] Epilepsy continued to be considered a contagious disease that could be spread by their breath, and to the end of the Middle Ages those with the condition were not allowed to sell food, drink from common water supplies, and were expelled from towns. In Middle Ages Scotland, men with epilepsy were castrated, while pregnant women with the condition were buried alive.[62] Epilepsy was again paired with leprosy as a condition whose sufferers were to be expelled from monasteries.[63] It would become apparent to me how widespread these misconceptions about epilepsy were when I moved to Asia. The Renaissance brought closer observation and description of epilepsy but little in the way of improved understanding or treatment.[64] It continued to be thought of as an infectious disease throughout the following centuries.

While this subsided some with the scientific revolution and the enlightenment, it would not alter the accuracy of Jerome Engel, Jr.'s, observation in his *Seizures and Epilepsy*, "To some degree in all cultures, people with epilepsy have been considered outcasts because of misconceptions relating symptoms to demonic possession, punishment for sins, contagious diseases, and insanity."[65]

By the 1700s there were many ambitious salesmen with elixirs and tonics that guaranteed cure of epilepsy as well as nearly all other conditions, such as Dr. Lowther's Powders, which, in the 1750s, were "a certain cure for Epileptic fits."[66] Unfortunately it was no longer available by the time I arrived in England. This would continue through the following century in the UK and the United States. One seemingly progressive offer came with the use of electricity, and the claim "It is very well known that epileptic cases, however obstinate and inveterate are removed and cured by the electric treatment."[67]

By the 19th century the relationship of mental health and epilepsy was well established as fact, as seen in a London *Times* report on a family's children: "One of them is in a state of lunacy from epileptic fits."[68] By that time even royalty wasn't spared public mention of epilepsy. It was reported in 1802 that Archduke Charles from Vienna suffered from status epilepticus, as "there was scarcely any intermission to the epileptic fits."[69] There would be incarceration in the name of humanitarianism for those with epilepsy along with "idiots" and the "insane poor."[70] This housing of epileptics with the insane furthered the connection in public understanding between epilepsy and insanity.[71] Later in the century there would be institutions for the incarceration of epileptics alone.[72] It wouldn't be until the mid–1800s that the belief in demonic possession was finally generally abandoned in the West, as the modern era in epileptology was introduced. Practitioners from then through the early 20th century considered epileptic seizures as resulting from two separate causes: an innate pre-disposition and a precipitating or exciting cause.[73] Heredity was deemed the major factor required in having epilepsy. The *British Medical Journal* supported this position in 1868, stating, "The occurrence of the fits is generally traceable more immediately to some special irritation, either of a mental or bodily kind. At the same time, it is my belief that the essence of the malady is due to a congenital diathesis, without the existence of which no amount of irritation could ever produce an epileptic seizure."[74]

The "exciting cause" that might bring on a seizure could be many things, but a common belief of the time was that epilepsy was brought on by sexual excitement or masturbation. Sir Charles Locock, obstetrician to Queen Victoria, published a paper in *The Lancet* in 1857 contending the compound potassium bromide was a treatment for epilepsy, and the first effective anti-seizure medication was introduced.[75] Potassium bromide had a calming, sedative effect and was seen as a restraint on masturbation and sexual excitement, enhancing its effectiveness.[76]

A modern understanding of epilepsy originated at this time among some physicians and scientists, the most outstanding being John Hughlings Jackson. At the beginning of the 19th century there were prominent scientists who believed the nervous system was under the control of the metaphysical soul. The debate between those with this view and others who sought a physical cause carried on into mid-century, but when Hughlings Jackson began his work on epilepsy he concluded it was the cortex of the brain that was directly related to bodily movements. Experiments were being done on dogs that involved using electricity to stimulate spots in their brains that supported his ideas.[77] Hughlings Jackson developed the concept that there were different categories of seizures with separate characteristics. He spoke of "dreamy states" and described seizures as originating from specific areas in the cerebral cortex, a theory that is close to present-day views. He also recognized focal motor seizures, localized partial seizures that produce jerking or some movement on one side of the body and are also known as "jacksonian seizures." In the words of leading epilepsy authorities Jerome Engel, Jr., and Timothy A. Pedley, "Hughlings Jackson, more than anyone, established a scientific approach to the study of epileptic phenomena."[78]

As the century came to an end there were people seriously studying the condition, while many were incarcerated for having an illness that was a disability, but a medical condition.

5

Useless Eaters

The 1900s began and those with epilepsy might have thought their situation could not get worse, but they were wrong. The emergence of phenobarbital in 1912 marked the beginning of an effective pharmacotherapy for the treatment of epilepsy.[1] Phenobarbital was the first medication I was given when I had my seizure in Morocco and I would continue to take it for a time after returning to the United States. There was now hope for controlling seizures and that was just beginning. Attitudes were not making the same progress.

Soon they would turn worse to a tragic degree. Famed author Jack London contributed to the stereotype of epilepsy victims with his 1914 book, *Told in the Drooling Room*[2]:

Feeb? Oh, that's feeble-minded. I thought you knew. We're all feebs in here. But I'm a high-grade feeb. Dr. Dalrymple says I'm too smart to be in the Home, but I never let on. It's a pretty good place. And don't throw fits like lots of the feebs. You see that house up there through the trees. The high-grade epilecs all live in it by themselves. They're stuck up because they ain't just ordinary feebs.

They call it the club house, and they say they're just as good as anybody outside, only they're sick. I don't like them much. They laugh at me, when they ain't busy throwing fits. But I don't care. I never have to be scared about falling down and busting my head. Sometimes they run around in circles trying to find a place to sit down quick, only they don't. Low-grade epilecs are disgusting, and high-grade epilecs put on airs. I'm glad I ain't an epilec. There ain't anything to them. They just talk big, that's all.[3]

What would be tragic for epilepsy victims would be the eugenics movement. Eugenics was born in England in the late 19th century after the rediscovery of Mendel's work on dominant and recessive traits in the heredity of beans, and Charles Darwin's cousin, Sir Francis Galton, invented the word.[4] To Galton it was the science of improving human heredity as was being done with livestock breeding, by encouraging the breeding of the best of human specimens and discouraging the breeding of others. To accomplish this, they assigned everyone to racial categories and each of these races was asserted to have both biological and

social characteristics. The belief was that just as Mendel had demonstrated how to breed beans, it was possible to breed humans for intellectual and socially desirable qualities. It also followed the appearances of
being scientific and put everything in a taxonomy, or hierarchy since the
purpose was to promote the breeding of a superior gene pool.

At the very base of that taxonomy sat the useless disabled, including those with epilepsy, who only take and never contribute. In England,
the idea gained a following especially among the elite, including Win-
ston Churchill,[5] then soon spread to America, where it seemed in tune
with Progressive Era thought of the time on applying science to create
a better society. Followers included among others President Theodore
Roosevelt, who said, "society has no business to permit degenerates
to reproduce their kind,"[6] and Woodrow Wilson, who signed the law
that allowed involuntary sterilization of epileptics and other undesirables when he was governor of New Jersey.[7] The Rockefeller Foundation
and the Carnegie Institution along with other philanthropic organizations funded eugenics studies[8] and courses on it were taught at Harvard,
Stanford, Yale and Princeton. By 1928 there were 376 American colleges
with courses dedicated to eugenics.[9]

The Eugenics Records Office at Cold Spring Harbor in Long Island,
New York, was the first organized staff to collect eugenic information
in the United States in an organized, formal manner.[10] Soon California
became the epicenter of the movement.[11] Stanford president David Starr
Jordan advocated the belief that talent and poverty were passed through
the blood in his 1902 book, *Blood of a Nation*,[12] in which he stated "the
blood of a nation determines its history" and "the history of a nation
determines its blood."[13] Jordan's reference to "blood" was the eugenics
idea of "germ-plasm" that controlled heredity.[14]

To save the germ plasm from contamination, states instituted laws
that required compulsory sterilization of epileptics, the feebleminded,
the blind, those with "criminal tendencies" and other undesirables. For
example, the Michigan statute stated, "It is the policy of the state to prevent the procreation and increase in number of feebleminded, insane
and epileptic persons, idiots, imbeciles, moral degenerates, and sexual
perverts likely to become a menace to society."[15] In 1907 Indiana was
the first state to adopt a compulsory sterilization law, followed within
months by Washington. Eventually 29 states would approve such laws.[16]

Pointing to danger down the line, a widely-used textbook published
in 1918, *Applied Eugenics*, stated, "From an historical point of view, the
first method which presents itself is execution."[17] A commonly suggested method for this elimination of those considered detrimental to
the future of the racial purity in the United States was public, locally

operated "lethal" or gas chambers.[18] Lumping people with epilepsy together with others considered "defectives" was reinforced following that. The *Journal of the American Institute of Criminal Law and Criminology* stated in 1926 that "epilepsy is consistently indexed under the heading of insanity"[19] and "even in the mildest types the epileptic shows the beginnings of a sadistic attitude."[20]

The following year eugenics reached the U.S. Supreme Court in a case that had originally been called *BUCK v. BELL, Superintendent of State Colony for Epileptics and Feeble Minded,*[21] but would simply be known as *BUCK v. BELL*. It officially approved involuntary sterilization of those with epilepsy and other "defectives" in this decision.[22] The case centered on the forced sterilization of 18-year-old Carrie Buck against her will while she was a resident of Virginia's State Colony of Epileptic and Feeble Minded, where her mother and grandmother had also resided. Justice Oliver Wendell Holmes concluded his opinion in the case with "Three generations of imbeciles are enough."[23] The practice was largely discontinued in the 1960s and state laws repealed in the 1970s, but by then over 60,000 people had been sterilized without their consent in America,[24] including an unknown percent of them incarcerated because of epilepsy.

Eugenics and sterilization were also popular in Europe. The Rockefeller Foundation helped found the German eugenics program and funded a program that included work on twins by the infamous Josef Mengele.[25] Hitler carefully followed the American eugenics movement and quoted from it in speeches throughout his rise to power.[26] Charles Goethe, who founded the Eugenics Society of Northern California, also worked with the Human Betterment Foundation of California as they sent reports to Germany and propagandized in the United States for the Nazis when they came to power. He visited Germany in 1934 and his letter on the organization's influence was published in the year-end report: "You will be interested to know, that your work has played a powerful part in shaping the opinions of the intellectuals behind Hitler in this epoch-making program. Everywhere I sensed that their opinions have been tremendously stimulated by American thought, and particularly by the work of the Human Betterment Foundation."[27] By the time of his visit, the Nazis had passed "the law for the prevention of progeny with hereditary disease" which ordered sterilization for all conditions they considered hereditary, including epilepsy along with visual and hearing impairment, learning disabilities, mental illness, deviants and homosexuality. Between 300,000 and 400,000 were sterilized in this program, with the most victims designated as being feebleminded, having schizophrenia and epilepsy.[28]

"Useless eaters" was what the government called them. Their eugenics claim was that these people drained the master race while not contributing. The Nazis worked to indoctrinate young Germans that those with epilepsy were among them. This problem from a school mathematics book illustrates that process: "Careful estimates place the number of mentally ill patients, epileptics and others in (German) institutions at 300,000 persons. What is the total yearly cost of this at four Reich marks per person per day? Disregarding repayment how many new Marriage Grant loans at 1000 marks each could this sum provide?"[29]

The worst time for people with epilepsy as well as for many others with disabilities came a month after World War II broke out. In October 1939 Hitler signed an order authorizing the killing of people considered inferior, those who were "life unworthy of life"[30] in another government phrase. The code name for the operation was T-4 for the headquarters, and the executions were carried out in secret extermination centers. Nursing homes and government run sanitaria were the initial targets and victims were bussed to castles, psychiatric hospitals, and other walled in structures. Initially they were killed by lethal injection but in 1940 the Nazis began using gas chambers disguised as showers in a precursor to the Holocaust. Following the executions, the bodies were cleared out of the chambers by workers and gold teeth were removed, then large numbers of corpses were cremated together. According to the United States Holocaust Memorial Museum, "Between 200,000 and 250,000 mentally and physically handicapped persons were murdered from 1939 to 1945 under the T-4 and other 'euthanasia' programs."[31] Again it was a terrible time to have epilepsy and there were many who didn't survive because of others' misconceptions.

The genocide of the Holocaust was seen as a final result of eugenic thinking and brought an end to its popularity.[32] That didn't make things fine for those with epilepsy who remained the "other." *Time* magazine began a 1954 article with "An epileptic living in Delaware is prohibited from driving a car, is branded a criminal if he tries to marry, and can be sterilized on the decision of community or state officials, none of whom need be doctors. His plight [was] duplicated to some extent in nearly half the 48 states."[33] In the United States until the 1970s when I developed my epilepsy it was legal to deny people who had seizures access to restaurants, theaters, recreational facilities and other public accommodations.[34] Prisoners didn't fare any better. The 1978 federal case *Owens-El v. Robinson* states, "inmates with epilepsy who experienced seizures … were routinely and inappropriately shackled to cots while naked or in hospital gowns, and some were held in these restraints for as long as 29 days."[35] Well into the 1970s, Iowa, North Carolina and Oregon were still conducting involuntary sterilization of those with the condition.[36] It was legal until the late 1970s in some states to annul adoptions if an adopted child developed epilepsy within five years of the adoption.[37] That was no longer the case in North Dakota and we were headed for a life overseas. Many advances in pharmacology and other treatment options had become available by this time, and I was about to explore them more than I could have imagined.

6

New Worlds, New Problems

I wasn't aware of all the history in the aftermath of being diagnosed and getting through my first two years with the condition, which seemed managed. It was August 1979 when we headed to Europe in search of last-minute teaching positions, knowing it might be a year-long break, waiting to return to our North Dakota jobs. At least we were going somewhere new where nobody knew that there was anything strange about me. My epilepsy medicine was going to be a problem if nothing worked out. Just before departing I had been given a prescription for 1000 Dilantin capsules of 100 milligrams and 1000 tablets of phenobarbital of 60 milligrams, so there was time, though I had some concern about crossing borders carrying that quantity of drugs.

When September arrived, we were in London and contacted E.C.I.S., a teacher placement agency we had signed up with months earlier. It was located in a London suburb and there was a message waiting for us. We learned that Professor Friedberg had been correct about schools being desperate when teachers failed to show up or left suddenly after arriving. The message said that the American School of Rome and the American Community School of London had openings and were anxious to reach us, since school was about to begin.

On the forms I had submitted to the placement agency I hadn't listed having epilepsy, and hoped to get a job before it came up, knowing what my chances were if people were aware of my secret disability. I had been aware of the stigma surrounding epilepsy since being diagnosed. We were hoping to begin a life in a new place where nobody knew us, and my condition seemed to be under control. I made a decision that many with epilepsy do when they believe they can pass, and that is denial. A British study found this to be common for people to attempt, being reluctant to report seizures to their general practitioners, since epilepsy affected their eligibility for driving licenses and it limited employment possibilities and social activities.[1] The stigma attached to having epilepsy can be worse than the seizures[2] so concealment has long

46

been a common way to escape.[3] Having epilepsy that others are aware of is a circumstance that can isolate and invite rejection. Dr. Orrin Devinsky, director of the Epilepsy Center at New York University, observed, "The feeling, for a lot of people, is that it does carry a lot worse stigma than a cancer, or an H.I.V. even."[4]

Stigma, which is the bane of those with epilepsy, is a word that had its origins in ancient Greece. It began as a reference to bodily signs, such as cuts, burns, tattoos, that ritually marked a blemished person such as a slave, criminal or traitor.[5] This association of "stigma" with brands or marks continued to the late 19th century, and described symbols used to identify and to punish slaves in the United States. Stigmas as symbols also indicated moral disgrace.[6] Since the late 19th century, stigma has described categories of people rather than individuals,[7] or as Ervin Goffman put it in his seminal work on the topic, "today the term is … applied more to the disgrace itself than to the bodily evidence of it."[8] He defined it as "an undesired differentness."[9] Goffman classified it more narrowly as "enacted stigma," which involves actual discrimination, such as that against a person with epilepsy because of their social unacceptability, and "felt stigma" which describes the shame of having a condition such as epilepsy and the fear of experiencing enacted stigma.[10] Like many others with epilepsy I experienced both felt and enacted stigma. It is likely the dramatic presentation of violent seizures and the inability of others to take any action that influences them contributes to stigmatization.[11] Goffman commented on the situation of those who attempt to pass and fail: "He who passes can also suffer the classic experience of exposure he is attempting to hide, by others present or by impersonal circumstances…. The epileptic subject to *grand mal* seizures provides a more extreme case; he might regain consciousness to find he has been lying on a public street, incontinent, moaning, and jerking convulsively—a discrediting of sanity that is eased only slightly by his not having been conscious during some of the episode."[12] His description of recovering from a seizure is familiar to those with the condition. Temkin reports that observing seizures has been so traumatic, that it has been known to produce similar reactions in "terrified bystanders."[13] Another category of stigma defined by Goffman that is known to all with epilepsy and a number of other conditions is "courtesy stigma." This is a name for the effect on people personally associated with those who are stigmatized, such as relatives and close friends. Goffman pointed out that this can be a double edged sword, writing, "The person with a courtesy stigma can in fact make both the stigmatized and the normal uncomfortable: by always being ready to carry a burden that is not 'really' theirs, they can confront everyone else with too much morality;

by treating the stigma as a neutral matter to be looked at in a direct, off-hand way, they open themselves and the stigmatized to misunderstanding by normals who may read offensiveness into this behavior."[14]

Though epilepsy had long been stigmatized and recognized as so, a formal method for assessing the impact on those with the conditions had been lacking.[15] In 1980 a tool was developed that provided a method for evaluating how people with epilepsy felt about the degree to which they faced stigma and how it affected their quality of life. It was the simple questionnaire that follows. On it, respondents were to answer on a 1–4 scale, where 1 was strongly disagree, 2 agree, 3 disagree and 4 strongly disagree:

Perceived stigma

 1. Employers I've dealt with have treated me fairly.
 2. People put unreasonable limits on what I can do.
 3. People who know I have epilepsy treat me differently.
 4. Most people I know are willing to be educated about epilepsy.
 5. It really doesn't matter what you say to people, they usually have their mind made up.
 6. I always feel I have to prove myself.

Perceived limitations

 7. My epilepsy is pretty obvious to people.
 8. Because of epilepsy, there is a limit to the things I can do.
 9. There is a good chance I could hurt myself during a seizure.
 10. If I get really nervous or tense, it can bring on a seizure.
 11. As long as I take care of myself, I can control my seizures.[16]

Following that there have been many more detailed and varied questionnaires developed. What they find is that the challenge of stigma is consistent. The most recent World Health Organization report put the number of people worldwide with epilepsy at fifty million and noted, "the stigma and discrimination that surround epilepsy worldwide are often more difficult to overcome than the seizures themselves."[17]

We were in London, so we took a train to Cobham, a village in the green belt surrounding London, where the American Community School of London was located. We were met at the train station and driven to the "school." Where we came from, schools were brick buildings with playgrounds next to them, so this was a surprise. The entrance was isolated by woods then a guardhouse before entering the grounds of the school, a 130-acre campus, which included a five-hole golf course, two soccer fields, tennis courts. Circling the campus was the "Rhododendron Trail," a beautiful, flowered path running through the woods. The school's main building was Heywood Manor, a massive, white two-story building, with wisteria growing on the sides and a large staircase leading to the entrance. Inside were elegant drapes and brass handles on the doors. Near this were several former outbuildings of the manor that had been converted into classrooms for the elementary school and the high school as well as the high school library that matched the main building's style. Scattered in were portable structures that housed the remaining classrooms, and a new two-story gymnasium with a viewing deck. The entire campus was all tended to and kept immaculate by an abundant staff of gardeners, so it was always spectacular.

Once we saw all of this our minds were made up. There was a grade four job available for Jane and a position for me as a middle school physical education teacher. I'd never taught physical education but they were willing to say my athletic background would qualify me since school was about to start the following day. Thus began my one year as a physical education teacher and our life in England.

We first found an apartment in Surbiton, a town that was a short train ride away, and I immediately needed to locate a doctor so I could refill my prescriptions and get the blood levels of my medicines tested. Locating the address of the closest clinic, I was taken aback. Had I wandered onto the set of a horror film? There was a corner lot with patches of grass, surrounded by a wood rail fence. In the center of the plot stood a small wood shack that had a plank across the front door. On the plank were hand painted white capital letters that spelled SURGERY. What a frightening thought. I entered, fearful perhaps I might be interrupting an operation being conducted by a handsaw and took a seat in the small waiting room. So I had learned that in British usage, surgery is a word for a doctor's office. I met the doctor and discussed my condition. He took a blood sample that he said would be sent to be tested for Dilantin level, and I was registered as a patient with National Health. I later pestered his office repeatedly and eventually found the medicine in my blood was in what was called the "therapeutic level," so it seemed there was little to concern me.

Living in England was terrific, though my father died soon after the first school year began. That would be one of the difficulties of overseas life, being far away from family. We soon settled in and enjoyed the cosmopolitan faculty and international students while we took advantage of the many things London and the surrounding area has to offer. When the first year was coming to an end, we decided that we were not returning to our jobs in the United States but would continue in England then see where else we might find similar work. On longer vacations we visited the continent, also north Africa. I also coached volleyball when school began and our first away trip was to Paris. Every year I would coach tennis which was usually held in Brussels for the season's final, and our team was included a local league with British schools that provided me with yearly tickets for Wimbledon. It was a happy time in many ways.

My epilepsy was not proving to be a problem, though it was a quiet and perpetual danger. There was nothing about me that indicated a serious disorder, which I had. Like many others with the condition when it is controlled, I was largely in denial. I tried to keep my epilepsy a private matter, out of concern how others would perceive me and how it might affect my job. The only people I confided in were those close friends who often saw me digging around in packets to get the correct pills to take, which required an explanation. All I suffered were occasional auras that passed without incident.

My treatment consisted of regular visits to my local doctor and once visiting a neurologist. They made changes in my medications, eliminating phenobarbital and adding Mysoline. Phenobarbital is a barbiturate, also known as a sedative or hypnotic, since from the time of its development it was used to cause sleep by slowing down the central nervous system. How effective it is at shutting down the functioning of the central nervous system would be made obvious to me years later, when in July 2019 Attorney General William Barr would announce an end to the moratorium on the federal death penalty that had been in place since 2003. Barr also said that rather than using the three-drug procedure that is commonly used, federal executions would be administered by injection of a single drug, phenobarbital.[18] Georgia, Missouri and Texas had already been using this for executions by the time Barr decided on it for federal executions.[19]

Going off something that would later be used to kill people was fine, but other drugs that could have similar effects would follow. Many were sedatives of some sort and had a tendency to cause some sluggishness. I had been a coffee drinker since junior high school but after developing epilepsy and taking anticonvulsants like these, it became more of a balancing act—lots of caffeine to offset the drowsiness induced by my medicines. They also divided the amount of Dilantin in half and added a newer drug, Tegretol, which was raised to 1400 milligrams, near the maximum the company listed. It was a large enough dose that side effects became a concern.

It is likely that anyone with epilepsy has anxiety at some point when starting a new drug or reading the accompanying sheet from the pharmacy that lists possible side effects. I've been on 15 different anti-seizure medications at some time and every one had a similar list of possible things that might happen when one started taking the drug. I was always taking drugs in combinations and side effects tend to increase at a greater rate than benefits when drugs are combined, which is why epileptologists prefer monotherapy, the treatment of the condition with one medicine. In over 40 years with the condition I haven't been on one drug except for the time when we first returned from Morocco before I was diagnosed. Tegretol, this drug that I was now adding, is really typical, but as a small sample of its possible side effects, the following are included: dizziness, drowsiness, disturbances of coordination, depression, confusion, speech disturbances, nausea, gastric distress, diarrhea, constipation, fever and chills, osteoporosis, hepatic failure, hepatitis, congestive heart failure, pulmonary embolism, aplastic anemia, bone marrow depression, impaired male fertility, testicular atrophy, aggravation of hypertension, pancreatitis. There are certainly some of these that would be apparent to someone and some cause death, but many might be attributed to or have other causes, so it is very difficult to isolate the drug and assign responsibility. I attribute some of my dizziness and drowsiness to the many drugs I have taken and over the years I developed osteoporosis, which was credited to extended anticonvulsant usage. But I have displayed other symptoms at times that show up on this and other long lists. It isn't clear. But is a person depressed as a side effect of a medication or because of having epilepsy? Often several medications are involved at the same time, only further confusing things.

One thing I was learning was that I was a good metabolizer. One doctor described me as a "hyper-metabolizer." Whenever I went on some new medicine, I seemed to need to have it pushed to what for most people are very high numbers in the attempt to keep my condition under control. Taking three drugs of varying doses three times per day was confusing and the practice I adopted then and have continued ever since has been quite successful at solving that. There are very small plastic bags one can get. I packed an entire daily dose of drugs into an individual bag which I could carry in my shirt pocket, usually making up about a month's supply at a time. Then I carried one bag with me each day to be sure I consumed all the correct amount of medicine.

As a teacher, I passed from physical education, to high school history, then finally department head and advanced placement teacher, enjoying them all. To accompany my being in denial about epilepsy I gained an incredible sense of false security, which seems to be a common correlation. I drove in conditions that one such as me should not have done, believing if I had an aura there would be time to pull off somewhere and be safe, even though that wasn't always true. There was no easy turnoff when I drove a school bus through Hammersmith Circle in London to get my school tennis team to a match, or followed switchbacks up high on very narrow mountain roads in Sicily where people honked their horns and carried on forward when rounding blind corners. But nothing happened other than auras. It seemed that if I kept quiet about things, my epilepsy was not going to be a great problem and would be my little secret in my life.

Still, there it was, just sitting in there, waiting.

We had close friends, the Fenskes, who had taken jobs in Singapore after our third year in London. They were very excited about the country and the Singapore American School where they were working, and they encouraged us to contact the superintendent, Mel Kuhbander. We did and he would be attending a large overseas teacher hiring conference that was held every year in London. We spoke with him at the conference and he confirmed that we would be receiving offers to come to Singapore.

The contracts soon arrived and I went in to speak with our London headmaster, telling him what I thought was the surprising news that though we had been offered jobs, they might not accept me once they found out about my health. I then admitted that I had epilepsy and he said he had always known about it. While that initially startled me and people had advised me to not mention it to him, even though we had National Health, the school's insurance had been paying for my contribution for prescriptions. My four years of secrecy had been indulged since I hadn't had outward manifestations of my condition. That was about to change in ways I could not have imagined.

We planned to head to Singapore, thinking it would be another four year stay before moving on to another location as we explored living around the world. It would end up being 31 years and the "black blizzards" residing in my head would soon come to the surface.

It was the summer of 1983 when we moved to Singapore. Singapore is an island nation that was a British colony and part of Malaysia until 1965. Its dense population is 75 percent Chinese and nearly 15 percent Malay with about 5 percent Indian. This does not include the considerable expatriate population involved in management of the many businesses working there and the numerous foreign workers brought in for construction and domestic service. It is located one degree north of the equator in Southeast Asia. This concrete jungle imposed upon a tropical rainforest is a small island nation where efficiency is paramount. Coming from North Dakota it was really a change to live in a country where the record low temperature is 69°. The temperature varies by about two degrees year round and the weather forecast for every day is for highs in the upper 80s to 90 and lows in the upper 70s, so when monsoon winds blow it is comfortable and evenings are consistently beautiful year round. The humidity is always high and combined with the heat, this proved to be a combination that was challenging for me.

Soon after arriving I found a medical practice near the house we were renting and went to see Dr. Selvadurai in the Pandan Valley Clinic. That was how things worked in Singapore. One saw a general practitioner and was referred to a specialist. I was referred to Dr. Nei I-Ping, a diminutive neurologist with a continuously pleasant manner and constant smile. It was a fortunate assignment. We conversed for a time as he took my case history and performed the common tests such as heel to toe walking, following his finger to the sides while my head was faced forward. He ordered blood tests and also used a tuning fork-like instrument to measure my tendon reactions, which were very poor. His report said I was having auras, or focal seizures, every few days but I hadn't had a major convulsion since February 1978, four and three-quarters years earlier. That was about to change.

We started our teaching jobs and continued to be active, joining a running club, the Hash House Harriers, swimming, playing squash at our expat club, The American Club. It was at the American Club that my long stretch without a major seizure was broken. I was playing squash with my friend Bob, and he handled it right. He didn't panic, but let it play out then took me to Jane to see whether anything should be done. I went in the next day and had my blood levels checked. My Dilantin came back above the "therapeutic level" and in what is called the "toxic level." That was a frequent result for me. It sounds a bit scary but it seems that it just increases things like drowsiness, likeliness of falling and other problems that I have from a variety of factors. On a Saturday later that year I was having a massage near the American Club where I had parked our car. I had a very violent seizure, and when I came to, I was sitting in a police car, being driven back to our apartment, which was embarrassing for all concerned. My doctor tried having me drop Mysoline and add Depakote to see if that would be the answer. It wasn't. While I was managing to keep this to myself, we spent time on an isolated island in Malaysia, went trekking in northern Thailand to the Burmese border, rented a van and travelled New Zealand from the farthest north to south extremes. In New Zealand we were spending time with a friend from our time in London and I had a tonic-clonic seizure, which frightened him. He took me into a clinic, and when I had a chance to see a doctor, the visit was brief. I first told him about my condition and that I'd had a seizure. The doctor's whole response was "You had a seizure? Isn't that what epileptics do?" I left and took a nap before we carried on.

During my first year of teaching in Singapore I had never had a seizure in front of the students. My aura would give me time to leave the classroom and usually get to the teachers' lounge where I could find a carpeted spot to get down on that was not near any hard objects. That changed in a small degree when I was coaching tennis. A friend, Don, had come to play against members of our team and I had a violent seizure. Don had called an ambulance and followed it to the hospital. There he called Jane, who met us at a local open-air ward in the hospital where I'd been taken, and she found it extremely upsetting. The other patients had been tied down to beds. I assume I had stopped seizing before I arrived, though perhaps they had done the same to me at some point. I was only there for a brief time then while she explained my situation and I was released and taken home.

Several years later I was with another teacher after school in the teachers' lounge showing a movie when I had an aura that wasn't stopping. I left the room and found what I thought was a soft spot on the grass nearby and laid down, ready for what came next. The seizure hit and my head snapped back, hitting the metal edge of a sprinkler system buried there. The beige shirt I was wearing that I was so fond of was soon entirely drenched in blood. I had a deep cut in my head that required stitches. The scar in my head is still very evident.

We had a major life change in the fall of 1985 and my epilepsy would be an issue. We hoped to adopt a child. There was a Taiwanese orphanage we learned about from friends in Singapore where others had adopted and we made inquiries. We went through the paperwork and home visit and all seemed ready. When the agency in Taiwan received our application, they approved it, but noticed I had mentioned epilepsy to the case worker who visited us. We were contacted and told that if our application was submitted to the Taiwan government it would be rejected, as adoptions to people with epilepsy were not allowed. They recommended that we submit a new application on an alternative form. This required a statement from a doctor that I was in good health, which my doctor who had originally referred me to the neurologist for epilepsy management was willing to complete. That turned out to be satisfactory and we went to Taiwan in October and met our two-month-old daughter, Anne. We went through the legal adoption ceremony at that time and Jane returned in December to pick her up to bring her back to Singapore.

Then it was of increased concern if I had a seizure at the wrong time, plus there was the worry that the time would come when it would be an issue about what she would think. Having your own daughter afraid of you or thinking of you as strange is something I hadn't considered before but it was an immediate reality. It would become obvious to me that having epilepsy was not only a stress I had to bear, but was also a psychological strain on my wife and daughter. Studies support the fact that this is often the case in families where there is an adult with chronic epilepsy.[20] I also knew people would be concerned for my daughter's safety because she was in my presence, which was another deflating reality. We hired a full-time maid, or amah, the first year following adoption, then a live-in maid for all the years following. That was a major difference of being a teacher in Singapore where this was the customary way of life, and both locals and expats had maids who did the cleaning, cooking, child care.

I had other experiences, and health complications emerged that may have been side effects of my medication. One that was unrelated was a lump that emerged on my face. It concerned me so I decided to have it checked in 1988 and the dermatologist cut it off. The biopsy result was that it was tuberculosis, which I hadn't realized could be located on the skin. After having my lungs X-rayed and finding they were not affected that was finished. Other problems emerged soon after that might have been related to the medication I was taking, which continued. My stomach bothered me and I visited a gastroenterologist who diagnosed me with gastritis. There were also metaplasia cells, which could prove to be a problem. Another thing I began to notice was a lack of feeling in my feet, which was diagnosed as neuropathy. It wasn't really troublesome at the time.

In 1989 I received a sabbatical to attend Harvard's Kennedy School of Government. Upon arriving in Cambridge, I immediately went to see Harvard University Health Services since medication would be necessary. There I had an appointment with Dr. Draskockzy, who performed a neurological exam and ordered a blood test. She immediately decided to make a dramatic change in the medicine prescribed by my Singapore doctor. She had me drop Tegretol and add Depakene, or Valproic acid, beginning at 1750 milligrams per day, for the purpose of reducing or eliminating my auras. When my auras continued, she upped the dose to 2500 milligrams of Depakene per day. We never had any discussion about what this might do to me, which according to the information sheet that came with the medication included numerous unsettling possibilities, but she found this dose necessary to get this into the "therapeutic level" on the blood tests. Those tests had my results above the therapeutic level for phenytoin, or Dilantin, another topic left ignored.

My auras were inconsistent but continued, then one day after class at the Kennedy School one persisted. I found a couch outside the classroom and tried to get comfortable then explained what might happen to several students who approached me to ask if I was all right. Next,

I have vague recollections of an ambulance and was taken to a hospital but soon released. I didn't see my doctor until two weeks later and after having blood drawn again. Her notes from the meeting indicate the principal topic was that I had a grand mal seizure and what my blood levels had been at the time of the seizure and since. She was increasing my Depakene, of Valproic acid, to 2750 milligrams per day and leaving the Dilantin where it was.

So my epilepsy wasn't a secret at the Kennedy School any longer, but people were not more distant or even really interested. At the school, I had one special class on using game theory to make decisions that was taught by Tom Schelling. Schelling was the foremost civilian nuclear strategist of the Cold War and while taking his course I decided I could teach it to high school students. When I approached him with that idea he asked, "Who would be better at it, Harvard graduates or high school students?" He was actually serious and we developed a friendship that endured from 1990 on. It led to my teaching a course based on his work, then eventually after he won the Nobel Prize in Economics for his work in game theory, writing books on him and his ideas.

7

There Were Two Men

During my early years in Singapore I was aware of the stigma attached to epilepsy there. I soon learned of others for whom stigma was a more oppressive concern. There were two special men, one I knew and one I knew of, who were involved with the country's most stigmatized people. The one I knew was aware of my epilepsy. He would soon get me involved with these people.

The two men were so very different yet so similar. One was a Christian white man and the other a brown skinned Hindu. They were of a similar age and grew up half a world apart, but from their youth they shared a remarkable similarity. While both were born where stigma, prejudice, and discrimination were assumed ways of life, each found those attitudes unacceptable at an early age. Both chose to side with those discriminated against in society that their families shunned as naturally inferior.

The man I only knew of was Devan Nair. When he was a 16-year-old student in 1939 on break from the elite Victoria School in Singapore he went to visit his family's Eng Kee Estate, a large rubber plantation in the southern Malay state of Jahor. It was a very uncertain time, as World War II had recently broken out in Europe but the fighting in Asia had been carrying on for two years since Japanese forces began conquering territory in China. Early after his return to the plantation Nair met Paramanan. He recorded his recollection of this first meeting with Paramanan and the events that followed in an unpublished memoir that his son, Janandas, sent to me after his father's death.

Nair's memory was "ebony black, he had the ugliest face in the world." Paramanan was a pariah, one of the untouchables, the lowest in the Hindu caste system. The name pariah was most commonly applied to Tamils, residents of southern India and Ceylon, now Sri Lanka, who had originally been brought into Malaya by the British as indentured workers for rubber plantations. Nair came from a high warrior caste from the southern Indian state of Kerala.

The initial meeting between the pariah and the high caste youth occurred when Nair's mother sent him to the estate's grocer. There, he told the shocked shopkeeper to serve Paramanan first because the pariah had arrived earlier. It was an incident this usually shunned man would not forget.

The news of what happened at the grocery store reached his home before Nair did. When he arrived, his mother screamed, "Go and have a bath. Cleanse yourself of the pollution. Otherwise you will not be allowed to take your meals at the same table with us." On Malayan rubber estates, they continued to observe traditional Indian caste distinctions. While there was intermingling among respectable castes, a line was drawn against the untouchables. The pariahs, being the lowest of the low, were isolated in separate labor quarters and were engaged in the most menial tasks. The staff on typical rubber estates consisted of administrative positions that were mainly Malays who with rare exceptions, tended to look down on and bully the Tamil laborers. Before the War, Tamil laborers were generally easy going, and put up with their exploitation as part of what they accepted as the natural order of the universe.

The Japanese joined Germany and Italy as the Axis powers and enlarged World War II in December 1941, with the bombing of Pearl Harbor and coordinated attacks on the U.S. territories of Guam, the Wake Islands and the Philippines, and the British targets of Hong Kong and Singapore. Those air attacks were followed on the same day by an invasion at the north end of British Malay, a peninsula, much of which was covered with jungle and at the bottom connected by a causeway to the island fortress of Singapore. No civil or military authority remained, and the Malay staffs on area rubber estates congregated for greater safety in Eng Kee Estate mainly under Nair's father's roof, since he was the most senior figure.

The British manager of Eng Kee Estate fled to the seeming security of Singapore. He left behind a three-month supply of rice, sugar and salt for the nearly 500 staff, laborers and their families on the estate and gave the keys of the estate storeroom to Nair's father. Nair's father knew lawlessness and shortages were coming. He feared looting and decided to remove the supplies to a wooden garage in his bungalow. While his concerns were for assuring safe keeping, his intentions were not understood by many of the laborers and there were rumbles of discontent that he ignored.

Two days after the removal of the supplies from the estate store to the Nair family's dwelling, the peace of a tropical evening was shattered by a group of pariahs armed with iron pipes, bicycle chains and chopping knives, who arrived outside the bungalow. Leading them was Paramanan. They stopped outside the gate, and Paramanan shouted that they had come to return the supplies to the storeroom. He ordered that the gate be unlocked, or he would break it open.

There were totally bewildered looks on the faces of Nair's father and the rest of the Malay staff on the terrace of the bungalow. It was simply beyond belief that Tamil laborers, and pariahs, of all people, dared behave like this. The senior Nair blustered and yelled, "Get out of here, or we will whip all of you." Paramanan nodded to his group, who began systematically to hack away at the gate. Within minutes the gate was in shambles, and Paramanan and his men stood inside the compound. Nair senior and the Malay men sat in stunned incomprehension while their wives whimpered.

Acting on quick intuition and to the astonishment of all present, young Devan Nair walked towards Paramanan and told him quietly, "Father removed the rice and sugar from the store only to prevent looting. But everyone on the estate will get his due share." Paramanan's face softened into a yellow-toothed smile and, to everybody's surprise, he said, "*Chinnayyah* (Young Sir), I would never accept the word of any of the scoundrels here. But I accept your word." He added that no one would be harmed and the supplies would be returned to the store and distributed fairly.

Every mark of subordination had vanished from Paramanan. It was a royal pariah who stood there. The higher caste members of Nair's staff crowded around and received their supplies from the pariahs. Two hours later, Paramanan came over to the Nair's bungalow with a few of his pariahs carrying three sacks of rations. There was not a word of protest from Nair's parents or the Malays about the supplies being polluted because they had been handled by untouchables. By this action Paramanan the pariah had emerged as the natural leader of the estate. An unspoken alliance developed between Paramanan and Nair senior, who came to rely on the pariah to ensure that the laborers did their work and carried out management's instructions.

Soon after, on February 15, 1942, Singapore fell to the conquering Japanese troops and Singapore was renamed *Syonan*, "Light of the South." Japanese military authority was established in a town near the Nairs' estate named Tangkak. Japanese officers came to Nair's estate and appointed the senior Nair as manager, responsible for order and discipline, and ordered him to resume rubber production with all previous staff and laborers. Rubber was necessary for Japan's war effort.

Within months of the beginning of the Japanese occupation of Malaya a new factor entered into the picture, the guerrillas of the Malayan

Peoples' Anti-Japanese Army, or MPAJA. The MPAJA was almost entirely Chinese in composition, and was controlled by the Communist Party of Malaya. One of the guerrillas had contacted Paramanan, through whom he arranged to meet Nair senior. Under cover of a dark night, two Chinese accompanied by Paramanan came to the Nair bungalow to speak privately to Devan Nair and his father. The guerrillas told them tens of thousands of "fellow-countrymen" were being trained and readied in the jungles. The MPAJA required whatever food and money the estate could spare. The senior Nair promised his cooperation. His survival required him to be in favor with both the Japanese and the MPAJA.

He initially kept his part of the bargain, since the Japanese authorities were pleased with the superior rubber production on Eng Kee Estate. They gave the credit to Nair senior, but those on the estate knew this was thanks to Paramanan, who was responsible for order and discipline. The MPAJA was satisfied because they regularly received a reasonable share of supplies.

Preserving the secrecy of arrangements with the MPAJA was a problem. It was agreed that they would approach the estate only through Paramanan, since it was not prudent that Chinese should be seen in a rubber estate on which the staff and workforce were entirely Indian. Paramanan would meet them in the jungle so that nobody in the estate would know. It was also arranged that Paramanan should not be seen in private consultation with Nair senior. Devan Nair became their contact person for the exchange of news and messages.

Almost daily after breakfast, young Nair would cycle to Tangkak, through a forest of rubber trees, and where the rubber trees gave way to coconut palms, toddy was prepared. He would make a routine stop at the toddy center, a shed beneath a rain tree, equipped with a wood table and a couple of rough benches. He would sit on one of the benches and Paramanan would provide him with a glass of fresh toddy, then they would exchange the latest news.

It took some time for him to break through Paramanan's deference before the high Nair caste. Paramanan wouldn't sit down in front of Nair or with him. When young Nair asked him why, he said, "I am a pariah, after all." Nair replied, "No. You are a human being like me, under God. Nairs and pariahs are man-made distinctions, not God-made ones." He added, "You can sit down before Gandhi, who is one of the world's greatest men."

Paramanan's eyes lit up and he asked Nair to tell him about Gandhi. That began Paramanan's very first lesson in history and politics and the lessons continued every morning for ten days, as Nair expounded on Gandhi, the iniquity of the caste system, the equality of human beings, human rights that Nair had studied in Singapore. Paramanan was visibly affected and above all, a born warrior had acquired a cause for which he would fight.

Building what came to be known as the Siam Death Railway soon became a major priority for the Japanese military. The book and film *The Bridge on the River Kwai* dealt with a very small section of the railroad and featured work done by allied prisoners of war. Little has been written about the thousands of Indian rubber estate laborers and Chinese tin mine workers who were shanghaied to work on the Death Railway, nearly all of whom perished. They were worked to death, or were killed off by heat, malaria, or malnutrition.

The Japanese conducted their shanghaiing operations by having about twenty to thirty military trucks suddenly swoop down on a rubber estate, and pick up every able-bodied male laborer for transportation to the Siam Death Railway. Nair and Paramanan visited a neighboring estate where this had happened and saw bereft mothers, wives and children grieving the loss of loved ones. Estate managers were first asked over the phone for the time of day when workers would not be in the field and in their quarters, and were warned that they would pay with their heads for any leak of information about the impending arrival of military trucks.

One morning in early 1943, the telephone in Nair senior's bungalow rang. It was a call from the Japanese military garrison in Tangkak that left Nair's father shaken. He said, "My God! The Japanese are coming tomorrow at nine in the morning to pick up our laborers. They want 75 able-bodied young men. What do I do?"

The senior Nair decided that he would simply have to keep silent about that telephone call. For young Devan Nair, it was also an acute moral dilemma because he couldn't think of a way to warn Paramanan and the laborers without endangering his father. Sleep totally eluded him that night. Which was the greater trust—the safety and security of his father and possibly himself, or the trust that delivered into his hands the lives and future of some 75 fellow human beings and their families? Which would be the greater betrayal, that of his father, who stood to lose his head, or a cause he shared with Paramanan and those who looked to him for leadership, the obstruction and eventual defeat of an evil tyranny? Something clicked in his head. The way was clear. He would pray for his father, and warn Paramanan.

It was pitch black when he crept out of the bungalow and found his way to the pariah quarters. He woke Paramanan and said: "The Japanese are coming in the morning with their lorries to take away our young men. Do what you have to do."

Morning came, and 25 Japanese trucks arrived. The Japanese were furious to discover that there were only old women and babies left. Everyone else had fled into the jungle. His father was astounded but Nair's prayers were answered. His father suffered nothing worse than slaps. His proven record as a successful manager for much needed supplies saved him his head.

Paramanan reported what happened to his MPAJA contacts, and Nair later learned from Paramanan that they thought highly of him. It was no surprise that a few days later, Nair was asked to do more. The MPAJA knew from Paramanan that nearly every morning Nair would cycle to Tangkak town to purchase groceries and other supplies. They asked him to stay longer in Tangkak each day, and record the number and direction of Japanese military vehicles, especially troop conveyances or what seemed to be ammunition trucks.

Nair obliged, and learned in due course that the information he supplied was put to good use by the MPAJA guerrillas. Several Japanese truck convoys were ambushed. Japanese casualties were high, and the counter-measures taken were appalling. Small Chinese villages on the fringes of the jungle, comprising mostly vegetable gardeners, pig farmers and so on, were raided. Their huts were burned and, in several cases, every man, woman, child was either burned alive, or bayoneted. For safety, the guerrillas were forced to move their camps deeper into the jungle.

Paramanan was capable of incredible callousness, like the cold-blooded murder of a Malay staff member of a neighboring estate, suspected as being a Japanese collaborator. Paramanan hacked him to death with an axe. Nair was horrified by this, and said it was "barbaric." Paramanan didn't understand the word and refused to recognize any alienation between them. Their cooperation with the MPAJA made their continued regular contacts inevitable, but Nair developed a sense of moral superiority that didn't seem to bother Paramanan in the least.

In the late spring of 1944, Nair was present when a Japanese officer from Tangkak visited his father in their bungalow to inform him that the Japanese authorities were convinced that some members of the local population were assisting the communist guerrillas. He wanted Nair's father's cooperation to spot and apprehend the "evil-doers" out to sabotage the Japanese war effort. Nair informed Paramanan about the Japanese officer's visit, and he alerted his MPAJA contact in the jungle. The resistance leaders in the jungle were not surprised. The Nairs were warned through Paramanan that there were increasing signs that Japanese agents from local collaborators had successfully infiltrated the workforce in several rubber estates as well as Chinese villages bordering the jungle. As a result, a number of raids had been carried out by the Japanese military on suspected resistance hideouts, and Chinese villages had been razed and villagers massacred. They were told to be extra careful about concealing their involvement.

In late November 1944, Nair spent time in Kuala Lumpur, then began a month-long visit to Eng Kee Estate. It would normally take only a couple of days before he contacted Paramanan, but this time there was no news from him or about him. Around mid–December a head laborer in the estate reported that he had seen Paramanan's horribly mutilated corpse strung up on a pole by the main road in Tangkak, at its junction with the lane leading to the dreaded Japanese Kempeitai, or Secret Police, office.

Nair and his father knew what this meant. Paramanan must have been subjected to every kind of gruesome torture the Japanese employed. These would have included severe beatings, burning cigarette ends poked into the flesh, fingernails pulled out one by one, followed by toenails. And if none of these tortures managed to persuade the man into revealing the identities of his collaborators, they would inflict the cruelest death imaginable. A favorite method was to stick one end of a rubber hose into the victim's mouth, the other end on a water tap, then turn on the tap. When the victim's bladder was full, his tormentors would jump up and down on his belly, so that the man's kidneys were fatally ruptured.

This could mean only one thing. Paramanan had not been broken. The Nairs were still safe and untouched. Still, Nair went to hide with his mother in a disused hut in a remote part of the estate. His father himself could not leave his post. Two months passed, and it became clear that the Japanese had been unable to force Paramanan to betray any of those involved with him.

It was mind-boggling, but the man was superhuman. They had not heard of anybody who had survived unbroken in spirit after the ghastly Japanese Kempeitai had set to work on them. Nair's father was incredulous and humbled. Nair was thoroughly ashamed of himself for his presumptions of moral superiority over Paramanan. He wrote, "To this day I am rendered mute by the memory of Paramanan. What price modern sociobiology? Indeed, what price all the pretentious know-it-alls in science, religion, politics or economics? I would not be alive today if my life had depended on somebody armored with a redoubtable doctorate in philosophy, rather than on an illiterate pariah." Any doubts he might have had about challenging innate caste superiority were obliterated.

Following World War II Nair became a teacher, which led to his involvement in unions. The British put him in detention from 1951 to 1953 and again from 1956 to 1959, when Singapore won self-government and the People's Action Party (PAP) came to power. He had become one of the early members of the PAP and in 1961 he helped found and was first head of the National Trades Union Congress (NTUC), the organization of unionized Singapore workers. He was elected to the Malaysian Parliament when Singapore was part of the Federation of Malaya, then elected to the Singapore Parliament after Singapore became an independent nation in August 1965. In 1981 Devan Nair became president of the Republic of Singapore, but with Paramanan's memory embedded in him he always remembered to look out for and respect the welfare of those who society rejected.

That concern for society's rejected people would bring him into contact with another remarkable man, a friend, the bearded and jovial Fred Gibson.[1] Fred was born in 1929 in Selma, Alabama. His father, like many other men in the area, was a Ku Klux Klan member. This was the heart of the segregated Deep South in the United States. In his youth, Alabama had a law against interracial marriage that carried a sentence of two to seven years of hard labor at the state penitentiary. When Fred was young the town passed a law against interracial play.

The incident that set him on the course his life would take came when he was nine. He had a good friend he played with regularly who was black. In spite of the new law, they continued to meet after segregated school and play on the banks of the Alabama River. One day his friend stopped showing up at their meeting place. Fred eventually ran into the boy's mother and asked where he'd been. She said, "Haven't you heard?" The boy had been kicked to death.

That was it for the young Fred, and later that day he was out on the road, hitchhiking as far as he could get from the vile place. He made it all the way across the country to Los Angeles before being located and returned home. Undeterred in his desire to escape his home and the hate that encompassed him, he ran away again, was returned, then he did it again. After he had run away repeatedly, the legal system stepped in and removed him from his home and he was incarcerated in juvenile detention for years. His escape from Selma and its strict segregation had not come easily.

Fred's strong ideas about right and wrong didn't change, and after he was released, he eventually decided to attend seminary. He began at North Texas State, but found the Texas Baptist Church "too confining." From there he went to Cozer Theological Seminary in Upland, Pennsylvania, in the late 1940s and Martin Luther King, Jr., was also a student there. While King was ahead of him in school, they became friends, and remained so. When the civil rights movement began and King gained national prominence as its principal spokesman, Fred was a preacher at an inner-city church in Brooklyn.

He was involved with the Reverend King and they trained students together for lunch counter sit-ins at segregated diners, instructing them to withstand taunts and how to fall without being injured when physically removed from counter stools. Fred and King carried on light-hearted banter while preparing volunteers to face hatred and bigotry, and Fred thought one of their conversations might have led to familiar words King later used when he said, "I'm not worried about anything. I'm not fearing any man." Gibson organized transportation for thousands to travel from New York to the Washington Mall in August of 1963 as part of the "March on Washington for Jobs and Freedom." There they heard one of history's most famous speeches, when the Rev. Martin Luther King, Jr., addressed the mixed-race assembled crowd of a quarter of a million people and targeted what was best in them, saying, "I have a dream."

King stated many dreams, and it was early in that speech he said, "I have a dream that one day this nation will rise up and live out the true meaning of its creed: 'We hold these truths to be self-evident: that all men are created equal.'" That was what was in Fred's heart. In 1978 he was transferred to Singapore's Baptist Church where he remained until 1994. There he met a new group that suffered greatly from unequal treatment, victims of leprosy.

These were the most outcast people in Singapore and it was concern for their welfare that brought Devan Nair and Fred Gibson together. Fred visited what was locally called "The Leper Camp" where active cases were contained and met the "people without faces," the shrouded groups that suffered extreme facial deterioration with collapsed noses, no lips or eyebrows and much more. They talked to him through a slit in their shrouds and drew away when he approached because, he believes, they feared doing harm to others. He also became active in the Singapore Leprosy Relief Association, which went by the acronym SILRA, and provided a residential enclosure for recovered victims of leprosy who were destitute and had been rejected by family and society. Fred served on the Board of Trustees of SILRA and took residents on bus trips around town with them so they could see their old neighborhoods. He took them swimming in the ocean after midnight when they wouldn't be stared at. He also took them to his church, but again after midnight, as he wanted it secret. Although some of the patients were Christians they weren't attending outside churches, and there were rigid members of his church who thought Fred was "not good to be around because he likes lepers. Might catch it."

President Devan Nair adopted SILRA as his official charity, and also became a member of its Board of Trustees. He took his role seriously and regularly came to meetings. Nair lived near the Gibsons and they became friends. At one meeting Nair said, "Let's do something special. How about a moonlight cruise? Go with this card (and he gave Gibson his identity card) and make arrangements at the harbor." Coca-Cola provided refreshments and the cruise was a success.

Nair suggested the patients organize their own social committee for renting movies and for arranging other entertainment. The idea was adopted and the patients rented their own bus and went to visit Changi Airport during the day, rode the escalators, and looked around. Gibson got a call and was told that the president needed to speak to him immediately. He was concerned and didn't know whether his green card was being revoked or what. The receptionist said, "The president will speak with you." Nair asked, "Do you know what your lepers are up to now?" He told Fred, then said, "I think it's wonderful." Gibson headed out to the airport to "herd them up."

Devan Nair was forced to resign as president of Singapore in 1985 for spurious reasons and he left Singapore. Fred Gibson remained and continued his work with the leprosy victims.

One thing Fred didn't tell me until years later was that he did contract leprosy in 1993. By then he had endured so many biopsies on his nose he feared it might collapse and asked to have them done elsewhere. He noticed that the feeling on his left side was affected and was suspicious. A doctor he visited sent him to a cardiologist who kicked Fred out of his office, and a neurologist confirmed what he suspected. From there he went to Dr. Seow, a colleague on the SILRA board and the foremost expert in Singapore on treating the disease. Fred was scheduled to leave Singapore and return to the United States in eleven months, and his fear was he would be incarcerated in Carville, Louisiana, the last remaining leprosarium in America. Seow prescribed the appropriate medicines and Fred said, "Give me all at once." Seow's response was "It will be worse than the disease," and he asked, "Can't you take it somewhere else?" Fred persisted and went in for a blood serum test after a period, where Dr. Seow told him, "You still have it, Fred." The results of his next test were that he was all right and the disease had been eliminated.

I visited Fred soon after he moved back to the United States. He was in his 80s and teaching in Spanish at a local jail along with his church duties and working with troubled goths, a counter-culture of an ill-defined nature with a preoccupation with death and often dressed in black. To the ever-uplifting Fred they were another group of enjoyable people to get to know.

I asked him how he always managed to be anxious to interact with those who many in society rejected and he said, "There's something golden and wonderful about every person.".

I'll never be Fred but I'll always be in his debt for introducing me to a very special group of people in Singapore.

8

A Synonym for Stigma

The old gray-haired lady had a distant and dejected look as she recalled the clothes she had been given to wear in her younger days. "We had a white kebaya and red sarong. On the left side of our kebaya was sewn a red ring. And in the middle was the letter L—'leper.'"[1] Peggy Arazoo had her own scarlet letter that publicly branded her as an outcast from society.

I first met Peggy in 1991 as a guest of Fred Gibson, where he had become involved with the people who were so stigmatized, their very existence had through much of history been a synonym for stigma. These were victims of leprosy. In 2003 the *New York Times* carried an article about a revival of cases in the United States with the title "Leprosy, a Synonym for a Stigma, Returns."[2] As *The Lancet* reported on leprosy, "The term has been so heavily stigmatized that it has become synonymous with abandonment, social isolation, and condemnation to a lifetime at the margins of society."[3]

Fred and I went to SILRA in 1991, as the Leper Camp no longer existed. SILRA provided a residential enclosure for recovered victims of leprosy who were destitute and remained outcasts. He was trying to convince me to bring students from the Singapore American School to visit the recovered victims of leprosy residing there. They were abandoned by their families and society and almost no outsiders entered their grounds. Having epilepsy, I was aware of people being stigmatized. Ignorance about epilepsy and stigma is longstanding and commonplace, and there are historical similarities between epilepsy and leprosy involving rejection that reach into modern times. With leprosy, it is of a different magnitude. Through much of history the situation for the condition's victims has been as Ethne Barnes describes in *Diseases and Human Evolution*: "To become a leper was to enter hell and damnation, to be turned away from family, friends, home, and all things familiar, forever."[4]

Before we arrived, Fred said, "You're going to like these people." He could not have been more accurate. The next year I began bringing students on weekly visits to the leprosy victims and continued to do so for the next 23 years.

Peggy died years ago and the labeled clothing is a thing of the distant past, but fear and ignorance remain ever present. She was recalling her days at the Leper Settlement in Singapore, commonly known at that time as the Leper Camp. After her years in the Leper Camp she had become a resident of SILRA, the Singapore Leprosy Relief Association Home, along with many others who passed through the Leper Settlement or Trafalgar Home, as it was renamed in 1950. SILRA provides destitute recovered patients of leprosy with accommodations and food, recognizing their exiled status from society.

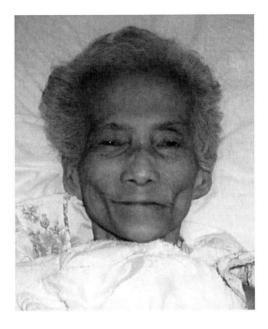

Peggy Arazoo shortly before her death.

These people there were "lepers," a group where their disease was their identity. I found that getting to know them and see the joy on their faces made life easier, and put whatever challenges I might have into a perspective that made mine seem trivial.

We began our weekly visits to about 140 residents on a sprawling compound with a small single gated entrance in 1992. There were rooms that could house four people, connected by walking paths that led to a central dining area where all meals were served, activities were carried out, and many spent much of their time. Attached to the dining room there were some rooms for the incapacitated, a workshop where several did weaving and some made baskets and soap trays among many items while others assembled paper umbrellas with labels stating "Made in Taiwan." There was also a small game room for mahjong and an office for the director. Overhead circular fans slowly moved the heavy tropical air and made it tolerable and helped keep some mosquitoes away. Dense jungle rimmed the back and a little used goldfish pool decorated the front. At first the compound appeared to our group a bit like an old folks' home. On many of the residents there was little evidence of having suffered from the disease, while visible deformities and varying degrees of damage were soon evident on others, such as missing fingers and toes, some collapsed noses or other facial damage, lost legs.

They were suspicious of us at first with good reason, as Director Francis Tan explained, since taxis had sometimes refused to pick up passengers, workmen had refused to enter to do repairs, and a reporter was going to do a story on them until Tan said he must shake hands with one of the residents.[5] We showed up only wanting to socialize and recognize them as individuals, but invaded the very sheltered and distrusting life they led. It was apparent that only returning regularly would make us accepted and we made weekly visits ever since when school was in session. In a short time, we were both expected and welcome. Residents could recall which students failed to attend on a Friday.

Soon after we began visits I made an attempt to shake hands with every resident on each occasion, tickled some and gave neck rubs to others when they were sitting in the dining hall waiting for dinner to be served. Soon some students were also shaking hands with many and the residents and Chinese speaking students were engaging some in conversations while several became involved in Chinese Checkers games. The barrier was broken, though several remained aloof.

These people had been rejected and had formed their own "families" of friends within the Home. They separated into clusters that constituted a social existence of people who made no judgments of them, while cliques and loners emerged and there were problems among them similar to other groups living in close quarters. Leprosy's stigma was different from others. Around the world, the belief about this most ancient of diseases that sets it apart from other stigmas is that it is seen not only a disease of the bodies, but of the souls of its victims.

Singapore is very cosmopolitan with its mixed Asian population that is considerably Westernized. Attitudes of many cultures are present and this is apparent in its history with leprosy. *Science* reported a DNA experiment on leprosy's spread in 2005 that described the consistency of reactions: "By Medieval times, cultures around the globe were familiar with the deforming lesions and decaying flesh that resulted in lepers being burned at the stake or carted off to die in remote colonies."[6]

Records in Singapore began when it was a British colony. The first effort to contain leprosy's victims came in 1845 with a poorly constructed house for those with leprosy and other indigents. A leper ward was added to one of the hospitals which soon became a series of leper sheds. In the press, there were calls for action, going so far as one published claim of it being "quite possible and highly probable that this direful disease has often been communicated to healthy friends who have unconsciously walked on the footsteps of a leper."[7] With growing Chinese immigration, there was an increase in the presence of beggars in advanced stages of the disease. The Dutch from nearby Indonesia were also dumping leprosy victims in Singapore in the middle of the nights,[8] further adding to its population. Island asylums had been set aside in neighboring Malaysia, and Singapore considered doing the same. After the nature of contagious disease was better understood, the Leper's Ordinance was enacted in 1899 that required an asylum and capture of leprosy sufferers. It was in an area known as Woodbridge near the Lunatic Asylum, where Singapore's "undesirables" were hidden away.

Leprosy is commonly related to moral weakness and sin. There can be little doubt that in the West, it is from the Bible that many people have derived their views of leprosy, where the disease is mentioned more than 50 times in eight different books[9] and described as a plague from God,[10] that those who have it were to be outcasts,[11] were "unclean."[12] In the New Testament on the two occasions when Jesus helped lepers, he didn't cure them, he cleansed them. Outcasts, unclean, a plague—leprosy was a moral condition as much as an illness. The biblical view spread worldwide with the spread of Christianity and no other disease conjures up equal revulsion or rejection. There is dispute among scholars over what medical conditions fell under the label of the ancient Hebrew word *tzaraat* that came to be translated as "leprosy." There is no dispute that the word "leprosy" is what appears in the Bible and has been taken as a reference to the disfiguring Hansen's disease that people recognize. By the Middle Ages in Europe those with leprosy were required wear special clothes, ring bells or shake clappers to warn others of their approach, never wash hands or garments in springs or streams, never talk to people unless downwind from them and more.

When he was committed to Singapore's leprosy asylum, Tan Geok Hong converted to Christianity and took the name Dominic. He remembered, "So, on Sunday, October 22, in 1933, my father brought me to the Leper Camp, to the home there, and when we were admitted there was one hospital assistant. My father handed him the letter and he said 'OK.' From that day there, in the year 1933 on October 22 on Sunday, I was admitted to that horrible place. And I stood there and I said to myself, 'It's just like a living death.'"[13]

"A living death" is a frightening observation, and one that has described leprosy throughout the ages. In Medieval Europe, the Mass of Separation was similar to a funeral for the living and was sometimes performed for victims of leprosy. Dominic came from a family with five siblings, twin sisters and three brothers. Since he entered the leprosy settlement in 1933, he was in government institutions until his death 75 years later. During all that time, he was never visited by a member of his family. He observed, "Because maybe I committed some sin somewhere during that time. But I won't believe all of that. The ones who got leprosy, we got fate, that's why we got this kind of disease. How did I get it? Once in a million. But that is a leper's world."[14]

Many places in Asian and in Africa have known it as "the big disease," because of the perceived damage not only to the body but to the soul and body of those it struck. On the Indian subcontinent, it was sometimes known as *Maha rog*, "the Great Disease." Indians often considered it a punishment for sins committed in a past life, and up to 1815 people with leprosy were sometimes disposed of by being buried alive.[15] Chinese have long considered it a punishment for improper conduct and the view persists. In China people with leprosy have routinely been expelled from villages and sometimes were forced into walled enclosures that were so wretched that some chose to take their own lives rather than enter. There were also periodic massacres of victims in China.

Chinese make up most of Singapore's and SILRA's population. Dr. Francis Seow, Singapore's foremost authority on the disease, commented on local attitudes: "Number one, the most common belief among the Chinese is that it is sexually transmitted." He spoke of one of his patients who was in his 70s whose wife had thrown him out of their house and refused to see him. She said, "He must have been having sex with some prostitute. The poor man couldn't explain that there is no way. The Chinese believe very strongly about that. And the other thing they believe is inheritance. You must be born with it. The children of people with leprosy are cursed in our society." Seow noted a minority difference: "Muslims accept it. To them it is God's will. We notice the Muslim patients of ours are very, very supportive. They will still look after their parents or children with leprosy at home; they don't try to distance themselves from them."[16]

Around the world, the response to people with leprosy has been to lock them away in isolated communities. That was Singapore's solution with the Leper Camp or Trafalgar Home, which was a prison, surrounded by a gate of high iron bars. In the early years of our visits most of the residents were like Peggy and Dominic and had developed the condition as children, been taken from their families and spent their lives isolated from the outside world at Trafalgar then moved to SILRA Home after they were considered recovered. Over time, immigrants and foreign workers with the condition were also moved in. At Trafalgar Home, there were 12 guards at the entrances to capture those who attempted to leave the grounds. Punishment for unauthorized departure was severe and those who attempted it and were captured did solitary confinement in small cells with bars. Trafalgar also became home and provided many with education and familiar surroundings. Peggy became a teacher for many who entered after her.

Suicides by those who couldn't face a life of rejection and physical deformity were common before effective drug therapy was developed. Opium use, gambling, prostitution all were Trafalgar activities. A fugitive who escaped from the police attempted to hide out at Trafalgar, thinking the police wouldn't dare enter the grounds to arrest him.

That reflects a common misconception that the disease can be transmitted by physical contact.[17] The belief was so strong that large leprosariums like Culion colony in the Philippines and Sungai Buloh in Malaysia issued their own money, so others wouldn't have to touch something that had been touched by a person with leprosy. Eugenics came to Asia as China and Japan passed laws preventing people with leprosy from having children, and in Singapore, for a time, leprosy patients were forbidden by law from marrying to make the disease die out. In parts of Malaysia during the 1930s couples could live together or marry only after the man was sterilized.

Though science caught up with the disease of the soul in 1873 that did little to change public rejection of those who contracted it. Dr. Gerhard Hansen of Norway identified the germ that causes leprosy, giving the condition its proper name, Hansen's disease. *Mycobacterium leprae* is a bacterium similar to tuberculosis, but the damage it does is mainly to the peripheral nerves, those nerves outside the brain and spinal cord. Leprosy itself is not a life-threatening condition and ranks as one of the least communicable of diseases. Ninety-five percent of people exposed to it have natural immunity, and not all forms of leprosy are considered contagious. It might be confined to patches on the skin and loss of feeling in hands and feet, as nerve damage eliminates effective transmission of signals. More severe forms lead to the greatest deformities and victims have nodules and patches on their faces, often collapsed nose bridges and may have thickened and wrinkled nose and forehead. Eyes can be affected to the point of blindness. In all cases, the loss of sensation in the hands and feet can lead to ulceration and infections from cuts. The method of transmitting the disease remains unclear, but inhaled droplets leaving one and entering another's upper respiratory tract is a common idea.

The first symptom of the disease is usually light-colored numb patches on the skin. The strength of the person's immune system dictates the course the disease takes, if left untreated. Chia Pua Song was a SILRA resident born in China in 1927. He came to Singapore after his father died when he was three, and he recalls being "about 4, 5, 6 years old," when he first discovered having the telltale patches. "My aunt, one day, when we were eating dinner, I haven't taken a shower, I used towel to wrap myself, and there is a red mark. She asked me how come your leg is like that. After two to three years, gradually, I found something wrong with my fingers. The flesh on my fingers disappeared."[18] The responses people get to the signs of the condition remain constant, in spite of it having an outpatient treatment that cures it since the 1980s.

Nerve damage sometimes leads to atrophy resulting from muscle weakness and deterioration. That can result in clawed fingers or "drop foot" deformities. Lim KAhLee, who is really Lim AhLee, was in Singapore institutions for leprosy patients and those who have recovered from leprosy from 1948. The confusion over his name is that he was the second of two Lim AhLees admitted in 1948, so he was assigned a new name for easier administration. Both men personally went by AhLee. He recalled before passing, "I have ulcer and drop foot and the ankles of both feet ruptured and the doctors told me the best thing to do was to have both of your legs amputated one at a time. So, I had my first operation in 1959 and the second one followed in a few years. When I first came in here I already had some deformities on my hands. So eventually my fingers became more and more clawed, and also been wasted. Although they are claw, I can still make use of my fingers to do whatever I want, with difficulty and inconveniences."[19] AhLee's mother visited him the first year he was committed to the institution, but his family vanished from his life after then until he died 68 years later. This is true even though he took up art and became a recognized handicapped artist whose work was displayed in Washington, D.C., and who was the subject of a television documentary and a local television film based on his life.

In all cases, the loss of sensation in the hands and feet can lead to ulceration and infections from cuts and burns. One result at Trafalgar Hospital was that it became common for residents to keep cats as pets, and the habit persisted to a degree at SILRA. Keeping cats around Trafalgar was useful since they kept rats away from fingers and toes or other skin that could be gnawed on unfelt while someone slept.

It has been the deformities that have characterized leprosy over the years, and there is no longer any reason for them to come about. With treatment, the condition is quickly cured before damage is done. This makes early identification all the more important. Some recalled the days before effective treatment was available. Lim Tai Cheng came to Singapore from China with his mother when he was a child before World War II and didn't get sick until he was a teenager. He was a basket weaver who appeared younger than he was up to his surprising death.

His symptoms weren't apparent to an outside observer, as he said, "You can see right, all those people, when they get sick, they lose their limbs just like that; fingers, toes. Before 1955, because there is no medicine, people couldn't help but lose their body parts. Some people couldn't do nothing else but watch their bodies rot, eat away at themselves."[20] Dominic described one: "I remember one kid in the Home, at that time there's no medicine, and lip was affected, closed up until only one hole. So, he couldn't take drinks and there were no straws. In the olden days, 1935, 1936, at that time, there was no straws. So, they used to come with paper or something and pour something inside the mouth. Within one month, he passed away."[21]

Leprosy has been dealt with only by isolating its victims in many cases throughout the years and waiting for them to die. A medical treatment, the oil of the chaulmoogra nut has a long history of use in Asia, where it appears in ancient Hindu writings about Rama and in Burmese folklore as a treatment for leprosy. Treatment with the oil could be topical or oral, but was very difficult to tolerate when swallowed, which limited its effectiveness. It was introduced to the West in the mid–19th century by a British doctor serving in the Indian Medical Service as a professor at the Bengal Medical College. From London, it spread to become the standard treatment worldwide, improved in the early 20th century when it was developed as an injection. Patients at SILRA recalled the unpleasantness of swallowing and the frequency of the injections with bitter memories, as new spots on battered flesh that turned leathery from abuse were sought for more jabs. This was how the Trafalgar residents were treated prior to World War II, and when Japan occupied Singapore things got worse.

World War II was especially difficult for the Singapore inmates. Before the Japanese came in 1942, they had doctors and food. During occupation, "the Japanese did not know what to do with us,"[22] recalled Lee Kiat Leng. He said they were completely locked in and isolated and the doctors and nurses taken away. The patients were left untreated and there were many deaths, not due to leprosy. They were provided very little food, and many weak patients died of hunger. Dominique adds they were given meat with maggots once daily or fish that had gone black and a small amount of rice. He contended that half the inmates of the Leper Colony died between the time the Japanese took control in 1942 and the British regained control in 1945. It was during the 1940s that the drug Dapsone was developed at the leprosarium Carville in Louisiana, and by the 1950s it was in widespread and effective use controlling leprosy. In the 1970s when it was apparent people were developing resistance to Dapsone, the World Health Organization began to recommend a combination of three drugs, and by the 1980s a multi-drug therapy was standard. It remains the standard treatment and cures the condition in six months to a year or more, making early detection especially important.

As the years passed I watched disease and old age thin the numbers of leprosy patients at SILRA. What started as 140 when I began was 39 when I moved on 23 years later and 35 when I visited Singapore recently. Many of those who remain had entered the Home since I first arrived, as the original residents had been reduced to a handful. I traveled with them both on day and overnight trips in Singapore and Malaysia. On these occasions, I found myself feeling very defensive when we entered shopping centers, markets and temples and watched for people's reactions in case any might cause humiliation or hints of rejection.

They were very special friends and I couldn't visit and not leave feeling better. These visits came at the end of the day on Friday when school was finished for the week and often I and the others who attended were run down from the week's demands. Then spending this time with these people meant one immediately abandoned petty concerns that had seemed important. I never learned Chinese so my interaction was mainly nonverbal, though some residents spoke some English. One, whom I often tickled and sometimes butted heads with, began calling me "monkey" one day when he gave me a banana, and he continued that for more than ten years. He had epilepsy as well as leprosy and I showed him my Dilantin which he also took to encourage him to take his more regularly, as he had seizures several times when I was present. For the students, this has also been a meaningful experience, not only interacting with the most stigmatized people but also becoming their friends then finding someone they had come to know and enjoy as a person had died since their last visit.

There was some improvement in Singapore and several other groups made occasional visits to the Home as time went by and corporations sponsored events. Still, progress was slow. The attitude they face was brought home when a Singaporean wanted to take some of the residents out to dinner in November 2004, and attempted to make table reservations. He was turned down everywhere he approached. A restaurant owner reply that shows the attitude still present was quoted in the newspaper, "We are running a decent business, not a charity organization. Let's say it's just too inconvenient. I wouldn't allow them even if you pay me."[23]

In his late years, I asked Dominic how he handled the stigma of ostracism of the most extreme form, rejected for 74 years. His answer was "I got this four words. Did I ever told you? L, O, V, E (as he counted out on the stubs of his fingers). L, Learn to control myself. O, my double smile. V, Very often, my tears will flow from my eyes. E, Every day I feel miserable or desperate while I sits alone. When I see and there's no one here, I feel very, very desperate and miserable. And that is the four words that is always in my mind."[24] I tried (K)AhLee, when he had gone beyond 50 years without a family visit, and he said, "Sometimes I feel very angry, and also very annoyed."[25] But somehow his success and renown as an artist had made him an extrovert when he had visitors, adding, "I'm always happy, thinking of something that might happen to me some day. In life, you have to be cheerful in order

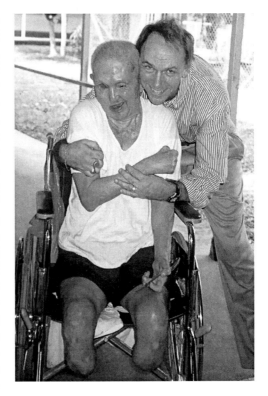

Author with Lee Kiat Leng at SILRA in Singapore.

to make ourselves healthier and stronger.... As the saying goes, laughter is the best medicine. So, I remain cheerful then I can be strong and healthy." He tried, but in his later years, depression got to him after his vision began to fail and his painting, which had been his escape, was no longer possible.

I'll always be thankful to Fred Gibson for introducing me to these people. I may not be better but I'm a wiser person for the years of enjoying their friendship. The leprosy home was going to hit me and open my mind to Goffman's understanding of stigma as a two-way street.[26] It isn't just a matter of how one is looked at by others; it is also a matter of how one looks at oneself. These people didn't view themselves as lesser or different, regardless of their awareness of what others' views might be.

While leprosy and epilepsy are always on lists of conditions that suffer from stigma, there are a variety of physical and mental health conditions where the term is equally applicable, as AIDS victims have been referred to by some as "today's lepers."[27] Many groups of people are marginalized by some form of rejection or stigma, and what I believe is that people only want to be seen as people, regardless of their physical condition or lifestyle choices. They experience the same emotions and react to kindness, condescension, rudeness, interest in them the same as others do. Whether they are transgender, quadriplegic, racially different or can't speak without stuttering doesn't define them. It is only a condition that is one part of a greater whole that gets overlooked once "we" forget to get to know "them." I should have understood that from my own life, but it took a group of friends from SILRA, Singapore's victims of leprosy, to make it really clear. I really liked those people, as Fred Gibson predicted.

9

They Don't Like Us Much Either

Making weekly visits to see the leprosy victims was good for me and kept what problems I had in perspective. After my first years of visits when the school year ended, we headed back to the United States for the summer and on the trip, something happened that everyone who travels and has epilepsy fears. The route we had begun using was to fly to Taipei where we had a layover, then across the ocean to San Francisco to connect with a short flight and be in Denver 20 hours later if things went well. That year we had flown to Taipei and boarded the flight to San Francisco when I didn't feel well. As we were taxiing down the runway Jane pushed the bell for assistance, but the stewardesses had been instructed by the pilot to be seated and fasten their seatbelts for take-off. That was when my seizure came. It wasn't dramatic and nobody contacted the pilot. A seizure was bad enough, but if the whole plane would have been turned around to take me back it would have singled me out for total humiliation. At least it wasn't in the middle of the ocean. Years later my doctor would give me a prescription for lorazepam, usually in the form of Ativan, which is a potent benzodiazepine he prescribed for "putting out fires." We discussed the use of it preventively in advance for situations where a seizure would be especially awkward or dangerous. Following that, I always took one just as I boarded long flights. That doctor was Dr. Lesser.

Dr. Ronald Lesser, Professor of Neurology and Neurosurgery at Johns Hopkins Hospital, would soon be overseeing my brain surgeries. He observed, "Leprosy may be a good example to contrast and compare with epilepsy. It is now usually a treatable disease—take the antibiotics and you'll do pretty well. If the cost of the antibiotics can be afforded, the main obstacles are people's fears."[1] When the World Health Organization announced its global campaign against the stigma associated with epilepsy, "Out of the Shadows," on June 19, 1997, its press release included the following statement: "Cancer, leprosy and epilepsy were the three great unmentionables until as recently as 30 years ago. Now cancer is more openly discussed while leprosy is less of a taboo, and we would like epilepsy to go that way."[2]

I wouldn't insult the people who had endured having leprosy by comparing the stigma attached to my condition with theirs. I was conducting what seemed like a normal life, while these people lived in an institution as outcasts in their own community.

What I had learned was that the acceptance of those of us with epilepsy in Asia was very superficial and extended as far as you could conceal your condition. The perception of people with epilepsy in Asia has had a long history of being disturbingly negative. This has managed to improve in only modest steps. Epilepsy has been written about in India in the *Ayurveda,* one of the four *Vedas* believers date to 6000 BC but western scholars put at 3000 years ago.[3] Though this work is not available in its original form, the treatise on Indian medicine *Samhitas,* written about 1000 BC, is considered the best representative of the original content.[4] This recognized four different kinds of seizures and presented methods for dealing with them that included mantras, or hymns, a wide variety of mainly herbal drugs which were to be administered as ointments or taken internally, blood-letting from the veins of the temple.[5] In China the earliest known document to mention epilepsy is *The Yellow Emperor's Classic of Internal Medicine* written by a group of physicians over centuries, beginning about 770 BC. In ancient times the Chinese identified five types of epilepsy.[6] Many different herbs were used for treatment along with scorpion, centipede, antelope horn.[7] While some of these traditional herbal remedies may have some anticonvulsive properties, none has been scientifically tested to a point where it would receive FDA or similar approval, and others tend to induce seizures while some cause problems when used in conjunction with modern epilepsy medication.[8] The view of those with epilepsy as reported by *The Lancet* remains that of facing persecution and discrimination: "In modern China, epilepsy generates a loss of face sufficient to make affected daughters unmarriageable, and leads families to hide patients at home, precluding treatment and control."[9]

When looking at Asian attitudes about people with epilepsy a place to start is the name of the disorder. I'd been described as having a seizure disorder or epilepsy. These names have been adopted by the educated and more cosmopolitan. However, epilepsy has many names in different Asian countries which indicate beliefs about those of us with the malady. In Chinese it's *dian xian,* which means "madness," or *yang dian feng,* meaning "goat madness."[10] In Malay, a language spoken mainly by people who are Muslim, the name is "gila babi," which is "mad pig disease." This is not only an insult but it compounds the stigma, since for most people who speak Malay, it names the person's condition for an animal that is religiously unclean.[11] The Cebuano dialect in the Philippines referred to convulsions as "boboyon," which translates as "pig gone mad," and in East Timor the term is *bibi maten*, meaning "dead goat."[12] It is thought that this is either because people sound like a goat when having a seizure, or because when goats are slaughtered they have convulsions.

Many languages of East Asian names for epilepsy are variations on the Chinese or Malay. Taiwan's and Hong Kong's are "dian xian," meaning "madness," the Korean word is "Gan-zil," or "mad sickness."[13] In Mongolia, epilepsy is "Unalt—tatalt," which is "madness, convulsion," while in Thai it is "Sok lom bai," meaning "sickness mad pig" or "mad pig disease." There is Myanmar's Burmese "Wet you pyan yawga," and Cambodia's Khmer "Chhkourt chrouk." These both translate as "mad pig disease."[14] With the Hmongs of Laos, epilepsy is the temporary disappearance of the soul out of the body, in a condition whose name translates as "the spirit catches you and you fall down."[15] This translation was the title of a very successful book on miscommunication between doctors and a Hmong family that settled in California and had a daughter with epilepsy.[16] When we lived in Asia I traveled in nearly all of these countries. The fact that people would have labeled me a mad pig, dead goat or any other of these monikers if they had been aware of my health is certainly unsettling as it no doubt was for many of the local residents.

Studies done reinforce the stigma and stereotyping of those with epilepsy in Asia. After I had lived in Singapore for seven years a survey published in the *Straits Times*, the nation's main paper, found the majority of the population felt people with epilepsy should be homebound. Dr. Andrew Pan, who was involved in carrying out the survey, recalls that only 30 percent of the population would allow their children to marry someone with epilepsy.[17] This article appeared shortly before Fred Gibson asked me to bring students to the leprosy home and influenced my willingness to say yes and reject the stigma surrounding them. In both India and China, epilepsy is commonly considered a valid reason for prohibiting or annulling marriages.[18] More than half in Asian surveys objected their children playing with children who sometimes had seizures, while over 80 percent believed epilepsy patients were unable to work the same as other people, and a similar number would object to their children marrying a person with epilepsy.[19] The divorce rate among people with epilepsy in Korea was ten times that of the general population.[20] In more progressive Hong Kong over 94 percent agreed that people with epilepsy should be able to get married, but just under 68 percent would be willing to allow their child to marry a person with epilepsy.[21] Asian attitudes appear to carry over in the United States with emigration, as a study found that the percentage of adult Chinese and Vietnamese in the United States who were opposed to employment of those with epilepsy was double that of native born American adults who oppose it.[22]

Singapore made some progress in attitudes during the 1990s. By 2000 about three-fourths had no objection to their children associating with someone with epilepsy while only 36 percent would object to their children marrying such a person.[23] Two out of five people said they would not know what to do if a person had a seizure, and while a third incorrectly thought that one should put something in the mouth of the person,[24] and one person's suggestion was "pricking the finger of the epilepsy sufferer till it bled."[25] A similar diversity of knowledge was displayed about causes as above 30 percent credited heredity, while among the novel ideas mentioned were eating goat's meat and the person having a black cat thrown at them.[26]

10

What Is Real?

At the time I began visits to the leprosy home, my own health problems intensified. I had a consultation with Dr. Nei on the morning of a work day in February of 1992. Following it I walked across the small street separating Mt. Elizabeth Clinic from Paragon, a large up-scale shopping mall on Orchard Road, to have coffee. Upon entering the building, I felt an aura that persisted. What happened next is unclear. It's possible I had a brief complex partial seizure somewhere obscure and no one noticed. I could have had total amnesia of it and might have managed to get myself up and then remembered my goal was to get to the coffee shop, though I would have been groggy and disoriented. It's also possible I had a brief tonic-clonic seizure that involved the entire brain in some concealed spot then came to in a confused state then realized my circumstances. I might have even made it to the coffee shop then had a seizure and attracted attention from management. All I'm certain of is that my wife received a call from someone at Paragon who said I was disoriented and carrying a large amount of cash. The caller wondered what should be done with me.

I was soon back across the street. Now it wasn't the clinic but the hospital, as I was admitted for observation. It was a two day stay and my doctor added a fourth drug to my epilepsy cocktail. I still had Dilantin, Epilim, Valproic acid, though the Valproic acid would be tapered off. The addition was Frisium, a benzodiazepine, which is a drug class commonly known for use as sedatives and can often cause dizziness and unsteadiness. It was not yet FDA approved as an anti-seizure medication.

This kept me in a condition where I would carry on with only infrequent major motor seizures and was able to be involved in most normal activities. In the spring of 1995 I went to Cambodia and saw sites that ranged from the splendor of Angkor Wat to the shock of the Killing Fields, with its 17-story stupa of human skulls and chips of bone fragments in the muddy earth on which we walked. It was a more shocking version of my visits to the leprosy home, as far as keeping things in perspective. My personal difficulties were trivial in the larger scale of things.

After returning to Singapore my stomach was constantly upset and I consumed vast quantities of antacids for well over a week, possibly the two weeks that followed. Whether that affected the absorption of my anti-seizure medication I'm unsure, but perhaps it led to what happened.

On a Friday in May I went out with my friends, fellow teachers, and we spent the evening snacking and drinking beer at the stalls, small stands that serve a great variety of local food. There were round marble-topped tables in the open frangipani and jasmine scented heavy tropical air where the crowd included the local HDB (public housing) residents as well as a scattering of professionals. Ice-cold beer was sold in liter bottles. It was great company and atmosphere, invited staying on until the stress of the week at school had been totally released, which that night required considerable consumption. I had been told many times about seizures and drinking but had never found a correlation in my case.

The next day I took my nine-year-old daughter, Anne, to the swimming pool at the American Club, where we often spent our free time. The pool was nestled outdoors between the Club's main entrance and neighboring properties, and lush foliage with a barrier of palms seemed to disguise its location in downtown Singapore. While Anne was in the pool, I was on a chaise lounge chair in the sun next to the edge. I felt an aura and as I often did when this happened at a pool, I jumped in to see if the sudden cooling off would help—perhaps not a great idea, but it occasionally seemed to be effective. Not this time, so I got back on the chaise lounge and waited to see what was coming. Soon everything went blank. I have no memories from this point on Saturday until Monday but my wife supplied the details of the intervening time.

She just happened to arrive and saw people gathered around and Abdul, a lifeguard, watching over me. I was stiff and unresponsive and they thought I might be having a stroke. Jane told them I was having a seizure and went to find someone to take care of Anne. Next Abdul, an amiable, stocky, short Malay, helped Jane get me into our car, then he held me as we drove to the nearest hospital. At that time, I began having seizures that continued repeatedly. Even though I was no longer conscious I was speaking incoherently, with the exception of saying repeatedly, "I've got to go to the bathroom."

I was having a status seizure, or *status epilepticus*, which can be life threatening. This type of seizure is especially dangerous if it becomes violently convulsive, as mine did, and a person must receive medical attention quickly if he or she is to survive without permanent damage or at all. What happens is the seizure continues without stopping and eventually the body and/or the brain gives out. These seizures are life threatening. Statistics vary but with emergency care the mortality factor is about 20 percent,[1] and increases with age. If not treated within an hour, the statistics given for adults of my age were that up to 40 percent will die. The journal *Brain* did a study of over a thousand cases to compare the effectiveness of different anesthetics used and in 2012 reported, "Overall, 35% of the patients died."[2] I could not know that this would only my first of repeated episodes.

After heavy sedation, my seizures finally stopped and then I was taken to intensive care, a shared room with a glass wall facing the nurses' office. My bathroom comments had been real and I had defecated during my seizures while on my bed in intensive care and was lying in what my bowels had released. I was naked and anyone walking past could see my humiliation. It wasn't embarrassing to me as I was still unaware and not in control of my thought processes. Jane asked if I could be cleaned and have a diaper. They cleaned the mess I'd made and after a couple of hours Jane had to find out what had happened to our daughter. Even though it was intensive care and I was attached to monitors that would have attracted attention if something changed dramatically, it was a shared room with patients separated by pull-around curtains and nurses who stopped in occasionally. When Jane returned, she thought there was insufficient attention to the precariousness of my condition, so she hired a night nurse to stay with me and went home to spend the night with Anne.

I was shocked when Jane told me it was Monday, not Saturday. It also upset me to learn I was in the Critical Care Unit. It may have been all the tranquilizers, likely diazepam or lorazepam, that had been injected into me but I was very nauseated once I became aware. Out of desperation I repeatedly stuck a finger down my throat in an unsuccessful attempt to make myself throw up for relief and eventually had my stomach pumped. I also had a probe in my stomach, an EEG, and learned a CT scan had been performed earlier. The CT scan showed "extensive areas of falx calcification." My hands and forearms were swollen and I managed to take several naps, during which my dreams were frightening.

Once I was awake, my perception was highly distorted. I heard Jane's voice with a heavy "Queen's English" accent, which seemed highly affected to me. I received punctures for taking blood several times to monitor drug levels and keep a vein open so more sedative could be administered in case I began convulsing again. When the needles were inserted, I could see blood shoot out of my arm then splatter on the walls and drip down. I demanded that my wife wipe the walls to clean up the mess, and I would try to clean it from where it had spattered on her face. I also sent her to listen to the nurses, since I could hear them talking about me. She obliged me. There was a clock on the wall in front of the bed and the numbers appeared to be backwards, counter-clockwise, while the minute hand was moving in the opposite direction from the second hand. As evening came and Jane was going to return home, I heard a thunderstorm outdoors and sirens, bells. Looking out the window and seeing sheets of rain, it was clear to me that the construction cranes were leaning and might fall. I was extremely anxious about Jane driving home and whether she would make it safely, though she and others later told me it hadn't rained that evening.

That night was when things were the most unusual and I wrote after being released, "I am not entirely convinced it was all hallucination." My recollection from the time was that I awoke at what appeared to be 1:50 a.m. but the clock was not moving. Since I was receiving medicine at regular intervals, I decided to buzz the nurses' station, which was across from my room and visible to me. I could see that several people were at the station and they were all slumped down and sleeping but their heads popped up upon hearing the buzz. One went to the room next to me then came to my room and assured me everything was fine, but I was convinced the night shift tried to get the patients to sleep then went to sleep as well.

This was soon followed by a series of visitors. First was Michael, a mustached Malay nurse. Soon after there was another male nurse named Michael, a blonde German who asked me if I spoke French. They tried to persuade me that the time on the clock was correct by showing me their watches which matched the time, but I was not convinced and asked to see a doctor. They also tried to convince me everything was as it should be, but it appeared to me that my IV bag was deflated and no liquid was in the tube. Eventually Dr. David arrived and also had me look at his watch. He left and I was asked whether I wanted something to help me sleep, but I refused. The Malay nurse Michael continued to assure me that his watch was consistent with my clock by having me observe the two for several minutes. I suspected that Dr. David had contacted someone to restart the clocks and wondered whether he was actually a doctor.

While nurse Michael was attempting to convince me that all was well and I was hallucinating, I felt my bed raising and lowering slightly. When another older nurse entered the room to try to control the situation, I commented on this, and it appeared to me that Michael stepped on some lever or similar device located on the floor by the bed, halting the movement. Once the older nurse left the movement started again and Michael insisted it wasn't happening.

I nodded off for a bit, but when I awoke, I saw someone digging through the gym bag on the right side of my bed that contained my personal things. I was confined by being attached to many tubes and could not do anything more than watch the person slip out, though I complained about what I'd seen later on. The nurses and amahs were pacing through the halls at this time saying "Good night" in a rhythmic, sing-song manner. I fell asleep shortly after this, but awoke to see the clock moving much too fast. The entire staff was going through a routine in which they continually repeated the same gestures and comments. I also had the impression all the clocks had been stopped and the staff had to move them forward to set them to the correct time. I sat up in my bed and watched and was noticed by a nurse noticed by a nurse at the nurses' station. She giggled and nodded in my direction to a nurse passing by who entered the room next to mine, separated by clear Plexiglas. There were a number of staff members in the room who all looked at me so I waved.

There was some confusion on the staff's part at this point and they decided to continue the repetitious charade. After a while as the clocks were being brought up to the correct time and were moving rapidly, some of the staff was getting fed up with the whole situation. One or two walked out and the language exchanged grew crude, as one surreptitiously directed an obscene gesture at me. As frustration grew, several more staff members walked out. This led others to do the same until most had left. However, a number didn't, and I planned to seek access to the checkout times of those on duty that night. Later, those who had left began to trickle back in.

I later learned that the hospital considered transferring me to the Psych Ward during this. When my wife heard this, her reaction was "Oh my God. He's losing his mind along with everything else." She called my brother-in-law, a pathology professor, who contacted a neurologist and was told that my paranoia was caused by the overdose of drugs for stopping the status seizure.

I improved some by Tuesday and from then until Thursday my hallucinating was confined generally to hearing music and sometimes experiencing rhythm, especially in my left ear. At times, I was hearing someone's television through vents. At other times, I seem to have converted some nonmusical background sounds, such as the air conditioning or the portable fan, into a sound with melody which was often chant-like. I had a private nurse for two nights and the clock was removed from my room. I managed to begin eating some food and my stomach was greatly improved. My balance was poor and I was aware of a numb sensation in my calves and feet. I was convinced that my poor balance was exacerbated by my lack of muscle sensitivity.

By Thursday I had several visitors and prior to that while Jane was with me regularly, she brought Anne by occasionally to cheer me up. AhLee, from the SILRA residential home for victims of leprosy where I made weekly visits, sent me a "get well" painting. He had taken up painting recently in spite of the limitations his lack of fingers presented and was on his way to becoming a famous disabled artist. I was surprised to have a visit from a hospital administrator followed by a gift of a bouquet of flowers from the hospital. That evening I was moved to a private room and Jane spent the night on the foldout couch before heading to work.

Colleagues from the high school faculty spent time with me the next day as I was not supposed to be left unattended. I had a physical therapy session with an extremely pregnant and friendly therapist. I was pathetic at the balance activities but had no trouble with the ball reflex testing. Following that I again had another blood test that frustrated the lab technicians throughout my stay. They had very difficult times locating any veins that would yield an adequate amount of blood, and would do repeated punctures, chase veins, often give up and ask for someone else to try after apologizing to me. This would remain a permanent problem that would only become more obvious as hospitalizations became more extensive.

Things were uneventful following that and while my head felt a bit fuzzy, I could walk confidently by myself. I was discharged on Saturday, which was exactly a week since I'd had my status seizure, and when I returned home I wrote up my memories of the experience. My concluding statement was:

Observations to date—I suppose this is the most frightening experience I have endured, and although I obviously feel better, I have a nagging feeling of distress, I suspect this is due to a number of things. I have some fear that it is all about to happen again. My head doesn't feel quite normal, which is most likely a result of the large amount and variety of drugs I am taking. I found the experience of hallucinating terrifying. The images were all negative, and I can't quite rid myself of them as of yet. I'll reiterate that the hallucinations seem to have taken place over a spectrum that ranges from the obviously unreal to the blurry status that merges into reality, and I can't sort some of it out. My memory seems to have faded about certain everyday things, like students in my classes. Other than the first time I was analyzed after returning from Africa years ago, this is the only time I thought I might be close to death, and it's very unsettling. I really hope something, somehow, is going to give me complete control of myself again, and let my daughter grow up with a normal father. Jane remains a tower of strength, and I often resent myself for being a burden to her in many ways. She knows just what needs to be done, and doesn't allow me to receive incompetent treatment, regardless of how she has to go about achieving her ends. There's no way I'll ever be able to repay her, and I know she would never ask me to, because her motivation is so unselfish.

I was 49 and this wouldn't be my last exposure to status seizures and hallucinations. While this experience was a new threat and I prided myself on rational thought, I gained a new understanding for people who do not distinguish external reality from the reality in their head. There is no doubt that my experiences were completely real to me at the time they occurred.

I had an appointment with my neurologist, Nei I-Ping, soon after being released from the hospital. He told me it was his job to put on a pleasant face, but he hadn't thought that I'd survive when my seizures had been so difficult to subdue and with the complications that followed. The seizure medications he had me on by this point included an increased dose of 600 milligrams of Dilantin per day, 2400 milligrams of Epilim, and small doses of Frisium and Lamictal. He also said he felt my case was too complicated for him. His specialty was stroke and he recommended I see Dr. Lim at Singapore General Hospital who was really an epilepsy specialist. I agreed to make an appointment with Dr. Lim, but it would be after we returned from the United States and summer vacation.

We headed to Colorado in early June to spend the summer high in Rocky National Park Mountain in Colorado at a cabin owned by my sister and her husband, which was our habit. Denver and Boulder were near and I managed appointments for consultations. First, I had an appointment with a neurologist in Boulder. He did an exam and said I still had "mild facial asymmetry, as well as mild cognitive impairment" from my status seizure. I also had unsteadiness that he thought could be attributed to my toxic level of Dilantin. In spite of that observation, his recommendation was that I keep my Dilantin level where it was and increase my Lamictal dose.

He recommended tests, including a nerve conduction test that confirmed I had a lack of sensation in my lower legs. Since no causes showed up in tests, he said I should give up alcohol for six months to see if that was what had brought it on. That was a real approach-avoidance conflict. Since the neuropathy was an irritation and I'd hoped to find a way to rid myself of it, finding the cause was something I desired. But if I found the cause was drinking, I wasn't sure I wanted to know, since it would mean an end to having a beer with friends or a glass of wine with a nice meal. So I was alcohol free for the next six months and it would turn out to make no difference.

A productive contact came thanks to my sister. Her PhD was in marketing and she had done volunteer work for the epilepsy community to help them in fundraising. Through this she had become a friend of Dr. Timothy Pedley, who had been national president of the American Epilepsy Society and the Epilepsy Foundation of America while based at Columbia University. He would also become the president of the American Association of Neurology and I'd been told that he was the foremost authority on epilepsy medications. My sister contacted him and sent him my information from Singapore. Pedley wrote to her, then he called me to discuss medication. His comment on Nei I-Ping's recommendation that I transition to Tegretol and Lamictal was "This may not be unreasonable." When we spoke, he said that in the fall he'd be in Singapore and could see me, and recommended I see one of two doctors in Denver he had trained. He added that none of his patients was on four different medicines like I was, and the few on three had severe seizures or were mentally retarded. He also described how different drugs interact, and said my goal should be to push one drug to a high level for control. If it could not be achieved, surgery was a possibility.

Because of Pedley I managed to get a consultation with one of the students he had trained. It was very informative and I emerged with four pages of legal pad notes He said my goal should be monotherapy on Tegretol, and went through the qualities of many common drugs. He added that mine might be refractory seizures that are not responsive to drugs, and surgery could be a reasonable option to consider. He told me about status, and said I had an increased possibility of reoccurrence since the circuitry to cause it was present. He put the danger at a 20 percent chance of survival without treatment and better than 50 percent if I received proper care. This was one of those things that would stick in my mind as I would spend months alone in a mountain cabin for many years, especially after suffering several more episodes of status seizures. This doctor made a surprisingly accurate observation by suggesting that my status seizure had occurred because I had a second minor lesion along with my temporal lobe. It wouldn't be until I had a grid implanted directly on my brain that a second focus appeared, not in my temporal lobe but my frontal lobe. He commented on my neuropathy, saying nerve tests could be done, but all that could be gained would be learning a name, not a cure.

One thing I appreciated was his discussion regarding reliance on blood level numbers by neurologists in making diagnoses and prescriptions. I had found and would continue to see that neurologists often relied heavily on blood levels being in what was listed as the "therapeutic level" without asking about the reactions or other testing of side effects, discussing whether generic or brand name drugs are appropriate, letting one know what to watch for or inquiring whether any common symptoms are occurring. I suspect this is a common experience for those with epilepsy when visiting doctors. "You're the boss," was his comment. He said the numbers are much less important than how you feel, what you want, your regular habits. Drugs affect different people in different ways, so saying a specific number represents the correct level is no more accurate than saying all people should only have a certain number of alcoholic beverages, when for some, having two will be too many while for others, they might be completely capable of functioning after having four. In all, I thought my experience was a bit less of a mystery when returning to Singapore in the fall.

11

Desperate Decision

Upon returning to Singapore in the fall of 1995 I had my first appointment with the man who would become my Asian doctor for epilepsy from that point on until returning to the United States. He was Senior Consultant at Singapore General Hospital, Lim Shih Hui. Dr. Lim was the first real epileptologist I had visited, and his background was extremely broad, having studied both Chinese and western medicine in Singapore and the UK, and being trained at Cleveland Clinic under Hans Lüder, a pioneer in brain surgery for the treatment of seizure disorders. After he familiarized himself with my case, we discussed the possibility of brain surgery. He said I had gone through enough different experiments with drugs that he could say I had refractory or drug-resistant epilepsy. In that case, he felt brain surgery was a reasonable alternative, adding that studies showed it was economically advantageous, as the cost would be high but given the high probability of success, it would mean an end to paying for medications that would otherwise be a lifetime expense. I was convinced. Dr. Lim also gave me the option of being the second person to ever have this operation in Singapore. That really didn't sound good. Having someone still "learning" cut open my head and remove some of my brain seemed like something to be avoided unless it was a really critical situation, which this wasn't.

Before my next appointment with Dr. Lim I had contacted my sister and she had once again asked for advice from Timothy Pedley, the national president of the American Epilepsy Society and the Epilepsy Foundation of America. Pedley sent me a letter explaining the surgery and what I thought was a surprisingly high estimate of the likely cost. He also wrote that if I chose to have it done, he would recommend it take place at one of two places: at Columbia under his supervision or at Johns Hopkins under the supervision of Ronald Lesser. Dr. Lim was impressed by the mention of these names, as he attended international conferences regularly and he said Pedley was the "world's foremost authority on epilepsy medication." He had also heard Lesser speak, so he wasn't surprised that I was deciding to return to the United States for the operation.

I chose Johns Hopkins since it was near my sister's home in suburban Washington, D.C. In February 1996, I made the trip to the United States and on the 20th my sister took me to Johns Hopkins Hospital in Baltimore. After the initial admission process I was sent to the fifth floor for the first stage, which was being evaluated in the Epilepsy Monitoring Unit. This is a six-room facility where I was given a private room. There I had electrodes glued to my head for continuous computerized EEG recording. Along with this there was a camera for constant video surveillance. Next to my bed I had a button that I was instructed to push if I felt an aura coming on or anything behavior or sensation indicating seizure activity. Both the video and EEG were displayed at a central station which was perpetually monitored, so a comparative record of my actions and brain waves would be analyzed by the doctors, and so that someone could come to my aid if I had a seizure. The idea was to capture any seizure activity and try to localize the focus to determine what part of the brain to remove.

My first visitor other than the people getting me settled in the room was someone from the accounts department, making sure I could pay for my stay. Even though I came with a letter of guarantee from my employer that all expenses would be covered, she asked for the two credit cards I had and took the maximum on each as prepayment. Except for having all the wires stuck to my head, it was quite informal and with Johns Hopkins being a teaching hospital, I had a regular group of interns and residents stopping in and asking, "Any seizures?" while some attempted tests neurologists commonly do on patients during exams, and others asked questions regularly asked during epilepsy appointments. My sister took time off her very busy schedule to stay with me through much of this. I enjoyed the staff and Dr. Vining, who was my attending doctor that visited me twice daily until Lesser returned from a speaking engagement somewhere.

I was in the unit for ten days, waiting for them to get a sufficient amount of information and complete all necessary tests. It seemed to be one of those situations where you want something to happen so it doesn't. Much of the time I was just lying in bed, either visiting with my sister, playing chess on a computerized set I brought with me, reading a Grisham book a student had given me, or talking to the staff. Someone from the neuropsychiatric unit came by four times and did five hours of IQ and performance testing where I had mixed results. I took the Wechsler Adult Intelligence Test and my IQ came out as >99th percentile, so not bad for being one of the people who were still being described in newspapers as a "retarded epileptic."[1] Though it is true that epilepsy occurs more frequently in people who are described as retarded, or having IQ levels below 70,[2] research indicates that while people with epilepsy commonly have difficulties with education as well as social adjustment, those who end up cognitive abnormalities often had them predating the onset of their epilepsy, not because of it.[3]

Throughout all of this it seemed like a situation where for the first time, I was actually hoping to have a seizure but I didn't even seem to be having auras as often as usual. I was completely tapered off my medications as well, though I know this only from the hospital records. At one point, they decided to try provoke something with music, my trigger for auras and sometimes seizures, and brought in a tape recorder to play loud, screechy music. I didn't notice any unusual feeling or sensation from it.

While it seemed to me that nothing was happening, Dr. Vining decided to get a more accurate reading of the brain waves in my head by ordering sphenoidal electrodes. These are thin wires several inches long that would be inserted directly into my brain so they don't have to get readings off the surface of the skull. It was going to be a painful process, so the nurse gave me a shot of the pain killer Demerol, which I had never heard of. I passed out shortly after and when I came to, the room was full of doctors. Through woozy eyes I could see the blood pressure gauge that was attached to my arm, and my pressure was below ten, a single digit. The progress notes for that day written by an epilepsy fellow said the procedure on the right side "was mildly traumatic and successfully placed after three attempts," while Dr. Vining's notes said, "He had significant reaction to Demerol—became hypertensive." They had given me other injections to counteract the Demerol and let me rest a bit. It is probably fortunate that my first exposure to this drug took place at Johns Hopkins Hospital, as whether I would have survived otherwise is questionable. The injections I had that countered the effects of the Demerol left me with no pain killer when I had recovered and Dr. Vining said we should carry on with the tests. They had me open my mouth and the nurse used something that looked rather pistol-like with a tapered barrel, that apparently held, then injected the metal wire. She positioned it just above where my lower jaw hangs from my head, between the mandible and cranium, where there is a small spot covered only by muscle and ligaments with no bone. There was a repulsive crackling sound as the wire pierced the tissue so near the ear, and the pain was sharp and short. First one side then the anticipation of the other. It was obvious why there was supposed to be pain killer.

The nurse, Heather, who inserted the sphenoidal electrodes was very pleasant and had been good company throughout my stay. She apologized for "trying to kill me" after the procedure. Days later, upon my release she repeated that on the discharge form, writing, "Good luck! Take good care of yourself. You were the most pleasurable patient I've ever taken care of and almost made a goner."

The record of my stay in the EMU raises a very disturbing awareness about myself. I have said that I feel like a normal person and I have this view, which is perhaps a delusion to keep me from becoming depressed or to support a somewhat fragile ego. While it was obviously apparent I was different when having convulsive seizures, it seemed less noticeable at other times, including when I have partial seizures where I remained completely conscious and aware. The record of my EMU time gives parallel lists of the time, patients' behavior and EEG and a summary. While I thought I eventually had one seizure, this record lists nine events, three of which were auras and six complex partial seizures. The frightening thing is the behavior they recorded that accompanied these events. This list was extensive and included the following: "Begins vocalizing and having bruxism" (gnashing or clenching teeth), "Starts singing," "Begins singing," again "Starts singing," "Hums," "Begins singing but can follow commands," "Talking but confused," "Looking for phone but can't find objects in left visual field," "First there was a change in the pitch of his voice and then Mr. Dodge would begin to sign his responses," "Has intermittent head and eye deviation to left," "Cannot respond appropriately," "Eventually answers questions correctly but is confused," "cannot sing or add," "Head and eyes deviate to left," "subtle twitching of the right face," "movements of the head and eyes to the left." All of these things took place when I thought I was aware and functioning normally, also without dramatic EEG activity.

This was many years ago and perhaps that has been how I often behaved when I was unaware of it. I still have partial seizures and generally carry on in social situations until they pass, assuming they will go unnoticed. Perhaps that is an unfounded assumption, looking at my behavior in this carefully observed situation. Perhaps when I'm sitting in a coffee shop or somewhere I start singing randomly or gnashing my teeth with a confused look on my face and people just ignore me. I really don't know, though people have occasionally asked me whether I was all right for what seemed like no reason. Possibly I have unknowingly frightened or disturbed people whom I consider friends or acquaintances.

When Dr. Lesser returned, he became my attending and remained my principal epilepsy doctor following that point. My sister's comment was that he "looked like he came right out of central casting." A trim man with a full head of grey hair and high cheekbones, he had a confident manner that was reassuring. About all you can do when you are an epilepsy patient is hope to find a doctor you really trust and I'd found mine. Right away he was honest. When I asked him whether this surgery would work, he said there was one way he could guarantee it. All they needed to do was take the whole brain.

Lesser told me that the readings from the room, along with MRIs and EEGs, were sufficient to indicate a focus in my right temporal lobe. Before scheduling surgery, we would have to do the Wada test, technically known as the intracarotid sodium amytal test, which he would conduct. Like everything they did, all the horrific possibilities were read through in advance and I was required to give "informed consent" that the dangers were clear. I was wheeled down in full hospital garb to a special room that included large machinery where I was placed on an examination table, lying on my back. Several people got me prepared and one made a small incision in my groin, then inserted a catheter in a large artery. I could feel it moving up my body, which was eerie. This angiogram I had in me was injected with an X-ray dye in my brain to see how the vessels were functioning. Following that a second medication was injected through the catheter. This was an anesthetic directed to my left carotid artery in my neck, which reduced me to functioning only on the right hemisphere of my brain. Dr. Lesser entered and we talked a bit while he had me perform a number of tasks, such as reading words, remembering what had been said, identifying pictures, shapes and objects. There was then a brief break to allow the sedation to wear off, then anesthetic was injected in my right carotid artery and the right hemisphere of my brain went blank. Dr. Lesser went through the same tests on the left hemisphere as he had on the right.

The critical function of this test was to see whether I was a good candidate for surgery. Language was the big issue that was being tested. Since it was supposed to be localized on one side, they wanted to be sure they weren't going to cut that part out. I had other reactions. I'd often heard about right brain, left brain differences, how the left is rational while the right is home to emotions and artistic expression. It's a convenient idea, but even though I was operating on only my right brain hemisphere for a time then only my left hemisphere, I never actually noticed anything obviously missing or felt any difference that corresponds to those assumptions. The only time I remember getting a strange feeling came at one point after I had looked at things that I was told to remember. Dr. Lesser later returned to that and got to where I was supposed to tell him what I had recently seen, and I felt something more like anger at him. It was as though he was humiliating me, and I was taking it personally. I'm not sure why I was upset with him, as it was just frustration, since the name of what I was supposed to recall was in my head, but I couldn't get it out. Apparently, the speech part was anesthetized and my mouth would not say it. Perhaps I could have written it or pointed to it if given choices.

Enough had been learned and my speech was concentrated in my left hemisphere while the seizure activity appeared to originate in the right, particularly the temporal lobe. This was the best outcome for surgery without great cognitive risk. It was scheduled for May.

12

Cold and Alone

April back in Singapore didn't start well, with generalized tonic-clonic seizures on the 3rd and another a week later on the 10th. We headed to the United States well ahead of the surgery, in mid–April. My wife and I settled in at my sister's home in Bethesda, near Washington, D.C., while our daughter went to Denver to stay with my wife's twin sister, Judy. I had preoperative appointments and some time to relax. On April 21, we went to Georgetown to meet friends who had come from New York. They were staying with people they knew and had been our close friends years earlier. It began as a pleasant evening of socializing and catching up, since we had all left Fargo many years ago. I ruined that when I had a violent tonic-clonic seizure that lasted for seven minutes. I wasn't done. Later the same evening I had another, and it continued so long an ambulance was called, because Jane knew the dangers of status epilepticus and when the danger point had been reached. While waiting for trauma care to arrive, she felt it necessary to attempt some emergency treatment with the help of the people present. She had something available for this situation.

After I had been released from the hospital for status epilepticus the previous year, Dr. Nei, my first Singapore neurologist, had given me a packet of football shaped suppositories that were infused with diazepam, a drug used to stop seizures. He was aware of my travel habits and our frequent time on isolated islands and similar places where emergency treatment would not be available. I had brought these with me when I went to a Malaysian island with friends before this trip back to America, though they expressed little enthusiasm for volunteering to administer them once I explained where they went. My wife carried them when we traveled together. So, since I had gone into this long-lasting seizure and was convulsing randomly, my wife decided it was time to make use of one, and friends had to get my pants lowered to a point where she could insert it in me. Fortunately, I found less humiliating options for similar occasions since then.

That seizure ended after fifteen minutes, but I didn't regain consciousness for hours. No doubt I was sedated by the ER responders and somehow transferred sound asleep from that point on. When I regained consciousness, I found myself recovering at Georgetown University's hospital. There was the humiliation of having this happen in front of old friends, even though they knew of my condition. Still, what dignity do you have left after people see your body flailing constantly out of control? And what do they really think? Regardless of how reassuring and sympathetic people are, it is still not possible to wonder.

On the day after I was released, I had an appointment with Dr. Lesser, who increased the amount of Tegretol I was taking from 1200 to 1600 milligrams daily. He also moved the date of my surgery up to May 3, or an earlier time if one became available. I also had an appointment with Dr. Lenz, who would do the surgery. Immediately upon meeting him I asked him to hold his hand out. He seemed puzzled. I asked again and he stuck out his hand with his finger separated. I watched closely to see whether they looked shaky in·any way, and was pleased to see he was stable. He was going to be cutting into my brain and I didn't want to have any erratic slices taken. His report of our meeting didn't mention the operation, but was a detailed discussion of my seizures. The consultation note he reported was:

> His seizures characteristically began with decreased hearing and a buzzing sensation in the ears. He then chews, stares, turns his head to the left hand side, may have some arm movement on the left greater than the right hand side. In the Epilepsy Monitoring Unit he was noted to have a change in pitch of his voice and sometimes to sing his response to questions by the epilepsy monitoring unit technicians. He would be oriented for about 4 minutes and then develop twitching on the right side of his face. After the partial complex seizures, he is confused from minutes to hours. The rate of these seizures is uncertain, though he had seven seizures in one week in the Epilepsy Monitoring Unit while off medications. The partial complex seizure with secondary generalization occurred twice in the Epilepsy Monitoring Unit and four times over the month following. Generalized seizures characteristically last 5–7 minutes, a period of confusion lasting for several hours. He had a left honymous hemianopsia (that is an absence of vision on half of the visual world in each eye) and left Todd's paralysis after these seizures. [Todd's paralysis is a period of brief paralysis that follows seizures usually just on one side of the body. It can last from half an hour to 36 hours with it usually being completely resolved at an average of 15 hours. Todd's paralysis might affect speech and vision[1]] and, one episode of status lasting 3½ hours with apostictal confusion lasting four days.

WADA test showed no evidence of language or memory function on the right-hand side.

By the beginning of May, a high school and college friend of mine flew in from California, which I really appreciated. We tried to have a pleasant time with lots of jokes, a great meal. Then the day arrived. It was a cool May morning when we reached Johns Hopkins Hospital and I went through processing. After changing into my hospital gown I waited with my wife and some family and friends, crowded together in the small changing quarters. I attempted to be positive and the company provided some distraction, while everybody remained outwardly upbeat. Dr. Lenz stopped by before prepping for the surgery to greet us. My friend Bob grabbed his arm and said, "While you're in there, could you take out the part about the ribbon?" It was a long-standing joke between us since college, as the only distinction at North Dakota State University when we graduated was "With Honors" which required a 3.65 average. We both had averages above 3.64 and mine rounded up while his rounded down so I was among the honors graduates who wore ribbons at graduation while he wasn't. This appearance of being relaxed and cheerful reflected the character of those who were there to show their support, but the underlying feeling was apprehension.

A nurse arrived with a wheelchair. I bid a brief goodbye and listened to optimistic final sendoffs as the nurse waited in the hallway. A cacophony of thoughts battled for my attention before I entered the corridor. After saying what I hoped wasn't my last goodbye, I settled in the chair and was rolled on a quiet ride down the passage to a secluded area where I was left.

I was cold and alone, sitting in my blue wheelchair parked in the small entryway next to a blue plastic curtain. Through the opening, I could see the operating table in the middle of a dimly lit room with large flat surgical lamps hovering over it at angles. It was just me, sitting all alone and not sure whether everything was coming to an end and the epilepsy had finally won. Dr. Lesser made it clear that there was a two or three percent chance that I would not survive this procedure and went through many other possibilities that could turn out gruesome. Memory loss was a real possibility as was speech impairment, though hopefully the Wada test had given them reason to believe that wouldn't be the case. The only thing he seemed fairly certain about was that I would have vision problems in my left visual field, a pie in the sky that would not have sight. Just the idea that maybe I wasn't going to survive and was being given specific numbers, even if they were small, meant they were real. And what was I going to be like after they took out part of my brain?

Still, there was supposed to be a 70 percent possibility this would put an end to my seizures and that was a good chance. But sitting there alone in this highly air-conditioned spot while I was settled and stoic, inside me anxiety was bubbling.

After what seemed like a long time, but was probably only minutes, someone rolled me into the operation room. There were many people, residents, nurses to do the labor, and doctors for various purposes. I was placed on the table and covered with a blanket, and asked whether I was warm enough. All attempted to be pleasant as they put me in position and attempted to make me comfortable, adjusting lights so the surgeon's view would be unimpaired by shadows. Needles were inserted in my arms.

Dr. Lenz, my surgeon, came in with his face covered in a green gauze mask like all the others in the room, and he inquired to be sure that I was ready. At this point, there was little choice in answers. The anesthesiologist spoke to me in a gentle manner and I began to feel something warm in my arm. He told me to begin to start counting backwards from ten. I looked up at the light above me, thinking it might be the last thing I would ever see, and my counting might have reached six. That was it.

For the next seven and a half hours I was in surgery and I was so heavily sedated that after it was finished I was not conscious for some time. My family and friends were in a small waiting room along with a group that came to accompany another patient who was undergoing brain surgery in another operating theater at the same time. Someone came to the room to give occasional status reports and unfortunately, the other patient died on the table.

During my procedure, I had been placed on my side with a roll under my right shoulder.

My head was shaved, pressed and draped and turned 45 degrees to the left-hand side. My head was clamped in place with what are called Mayfield pins, so if I happened to have a seizure during surgery it would remain immobile and my brain wouldn't be sliced into strips before the surgeon removed his scalpel or the saw, if he was still getting through the skull. This clamp left marks in my forehead. The first part of the operation was to get the brain exposed and involved making a large backwards question mark incision through the skull and dura, the tough, fibrous material under the bone that protects the brain. He began this incision in front of the cheek bone close to the bottom of my right ear, continued rising up along the ear to the top, then turning back to the rear of my head where it curved up to the hair line and continued out to my forehead, about two inches above my right eyebrow. This was a long cut through very hard, protective material. Dr. Lesser had said, "It's a bit like carpentry," when describing the surgery, and I guess this is the part he was talking about. What the operative report described as a "five-hole free bone flap" was then turned back and this exposed part of the frontal lobe and right temporal lobe of my brain.

At this point they entered the brain and things became very

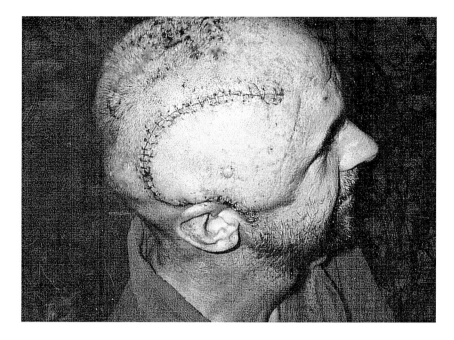

Staples to close surgical incision.

delicate. Dr. Lenz made an incision to locate the Sylvian fissure which separates the temporal lobe from the frontal and parietal lobes. He made his way through the white matter until encountering a brain ventricle, which he navigated using a hoop, suctioning and cauterizing. Then he made a number of cuts, used sutures and inserted cottonoid, an absorbent material, to reach the intended location where seizure activity had been identified. Lenz removed a section of the right temporal lobe, specifically the medial temporal lobe. He also took "in piecemeal fashion" the amygdala, a region generally associated with processing emotions, portions of the hippocampus, a seahorse shaped structure considered essential to learning and memory, and parahippocampal gyrus, which is thought to control many cognitive processes, including visuospatial processing and episodic memory. After cutting a bit farther, more bits of the hippocampus and parahippocampal gyrus were removed.

Once things were removed and samples taken for lab work, there was closing. An epidural drain was left since there was considerable cutting and resection so drainage would be significant. The dura was closed with braided nylon was left. The bone flap was maintained with titanium plates and bolts. The incision was closed with 40 staples plus nylon for the skin on the forehead.[2]

My first recollection since the anesthesiologist asked me to count backwards was the foggy presence of a room. As I gained some consciousness, I was very uncomfortable and only minimally aware of what was happening. I was beginning to realize that it was over but the sedation had only partially vanished. During the initial time in intensive care I didn't move and only opened my eyes occasionally. In my head and perhaps even very softly to myself I recited the words of "The Impossible Dream" from *The Man of La Mancha* over and over. It seemed helpful in convincing myself to hold on, regardless of whatever came next.

It became increasingly clear that I had made it and was lying there with half of my swollen head shaved and 40 metal staples outlining a large inverted question mark scar that started high on my forehead and wound around the side of my head then extended down alongside of my ear, holding my skull together. There was a drain for the yuck that was seeping out of my brain, as well as bruises from the clamp on my head, along with IVs in my arm for feeding and in case of seizures, as well as a catheter. I was not at my most attractive. My wife, Jane, was the only one allowed to come in for a visit during initial recovery, but seeing her was all I needed to know that I had made it.

When others came in I told my friend Bob, "I still remember the ribbon." My first question for Dr. Lenz after he commented on the operation was to ask him to name any date from 3000 BC on. He was slightly befuddled, but one of the others in the room came up with a random response. For me, it was a critical test, since I trusted my memory for teaching and for being able to start a class with that information. If I hadn't been able to begin speaking for 80 minutes about history from that point in time, then something would have been lost during the operation. I hadn't realized how much my memory was in the balance, as I was only aware of the temporal lobe being resected, or partially removed, but it seemed to have survived.

The whole experience had been a bit like an exaggerated seizure, with the panic of the aura taking place during the wait as I looked in at the operating theater and was taken and readied. Once the anesthetic was in me, I was out. It was total amnesia like while having tonic-clonic seizures. After coming to there had been a slow process of regaining clarity and I was very drowsy. Following violent seizures things were also confusing and it was also common for me to sleep for a time. This was on a much larger scale and I next learned why.

The operation had aimed for the area in the temporal lobe where the many MRIs and various scans indicated my focal point for interrupted brain activity was located. Dr. Lenz carved out an area around the focus and removed a fair portion of my temporal lobe in an operation called a right temporal lobectomy and amygdalohippocampectomy.

13

Anticlimax

Hope proved really fleeting. As I was being transferred from intensive care to my recovery room, I had a seizure in my wheelchair. My wife recalls the nurse saying, "Robert, Robert. Stop that, Stop that!" As if I had decided it would be something fun to do at that time? It was minor and I really hadn't noticed it, since I was still groggy, but it was certainly disappointing news when Jane told me. With that, I settled in to a private room for recovery from the surgery which would last 10 days. My wife was there throughout and my sister much of the time, along with other relatives and calls from friends plus several visitors.

For a time, I was experiencing what my hospital records described as "considerable nausea and malaise as well as lethargy." This was to a point where when my nephew, an Army doctor, and his wife visited. I made an attempt to leave my bed and get on the floor with IVs attached and crawl to the bathroom to put my finger down my throat so I would vomit. Though they restrained me, I made it another time but found that my finger only made me gag. The continuous nausea and the seizure took me farther. I got to a point where I asked my wife Jane to kill me.

The hospital took me off Tegretol, a drug that had caused me stomach difficulties since I had added it to my regime of epilepsy medications, and gave me salt tablets. In time, I felt much better and could carry on more normally.

During this recovery stay, I received many "get well" cards and flowers. Clearly the most special one came in a large envelope that was full of messages from the residents of SILRA, the home for victims of leprosy in Singapore. Some might think it ironic or embarrassing to receive get well messages from people who had leprosy, but nothing could have encouraged me more than these letters and notes. Knowing that these special people cared about my welfare was incredibly heartening.

There was follow-up testing to see whether the operation had done permanent damage. I took the Wechsler Adult Intelligence Test and the incongruous result was that my IQ had increased to 150, which was two points higher, by the removal of a substantial amount of brain. Things were opposite when I was tested for psychomotor functioning. The actual test involved timing how fast you could put small pegs in a pegboard. My score was < 2nd percentile so extremely clumsy. I suspect my verbal capability became for me something like what balance and daring had been for the boy Curt that I had known when I was young. He had done death defying things and I suspect that was in part to demonstrate to himself and others that he was not limited, not inferior because of his epilepsy, but was in fact beyond others in spite of it. It wasn't because of my score on this test, but since being diagnosed with the condition, as a defense mechanism, I defined myself with intellect to a certain degree, in what I taught, how I taught it, how I talked, my willingness to argue as much as discuss and to throw in extra information. I suspect part of this was also overcoming the side effects of drugs that made me slower, and I resented that and worked at not letting myself fall into mental laziness that can be part of the life of regular sedation. Soon after this I considered joining MENSA, not because it was an organization that did anything that interested me. I remembered that Stephen Hawking had joined after being diagnosed with the degenerative motor neuron disease amyotrophic lateral sclerosis, or ALS, when he was 20. I wasn't pretending to be at his level, but wasn't sure whether he joined just to prove to himself that he was still mentally functioning well, or to demonstrate that to others who might assume that because of his disease his mind was no longer what it once had been. My concern was that people already would make assumptions about my mental ability because I had epilepsy, and those conjectures would be compounded since I had undergone brain surgery and eventually multiple brain surgeries. My wife and sister both thought it would look arrogant more than anything else and were no doubt correct so I didn't pursue it.

Before I could be discharged there was another test of the ability to function on one's own. This involved a simulated kitchen where I made tea and toast, placed a phone call to order a video and had a conversation with two staff members. It was determined that I was in good enough shape to be released, and I was hoping the seizure that followed surgery was an anomaly.

I had been allowed a brief outing and went to Baltimore's Inner Harbor. While I was there, after strolling through the shops, I stopped for coffee. I was with my sister and a young man who had several body piercings stopped by our table to look at my head, then said, "That's cool!" I didn't mention that they weren't decorative. Soon I returned to stay at my sister's home and was pleased to be away from Baltimore and the hospital. One enjoyable moment was flushing my remaining

Tegretol down a toilet, as it had long caused me to be nauseated and made life challenging. Neurontin had been prescribed to replace it so perhaps that would work better. On my third night, there I was in the dining room about to walk into the family room where people were watching television. There was a tingling in my hand, my senses weren't quite focused so I stopped. It was all so familiar, but seemed like it couldn't be. I headed straight over to the carpet in the entryway hall, then down on the ground, still hoping it was something else. It wasn't. Though it was not violent, more of a simple partial or perhaps partial with slight twitching and jerks, it was definitely a seizure. This really settled that the seizure I had coming out of the recovery room was not a freak occurrence.

I had appointments coming up within the next few days with both my surgeon, Dr. Lenz, and my doctor, Dr. Lesser. Dr. Lenz was rather cold in his evaluation as he said that they had told us this operation works in 70 percent of the cases. That meant it didn't work in 30 percent. Somebody had to be in the 30 percent and I was one of those people. Dr. Lesser tried to be more uplifting, as he said it is not unusual for patients to have seizures following surgery and then become seizure-free, although they clearly preferred that this not occur. I pretended to believe his hopeful comment that I might be fine and seizures would become only a memory, but could tell he was disappointed things hadn't gone better. We then discussed medication, since with the surgery apparently having failed, my current medication was also not adequate. At the time, I was taking 350 milligrams of Lamictal and 2400 milligrams of Neurontin. He insisted I could tell the difference, which I couldn't, but I chose Neurontin, perhaps because of familiarity. He thought that was reasonable and I was instructed to increase Neurontin in 300 to 600 milligram increments every five days until I was taking between 3600 and 4200 milligrams daily. He said that I could increase the dose further if that became necessary, but this was a good place at least to start.

This illustrates the position epilepsy patients find themselves in as far as handling their care. One can do research and learn about medications, side effects, procedures, but what it really comes down to is finding a doctor that one can really trust. That is why I always insist on seeing epileptologists rather than neurologists and have been fortunate to have had outstanding treatment much of the time. Dr. Lesser was the person I had decided on as the one to trust and to this day I seek his advice before making any decisions. He was an expert on many areas related to epilepsy and its treatment. Then there was his suggestion about Neurontin. No doubt he had seen the drug used at the level he instructed me to use, but I never knew anything other than to take his word. A major manufacturer of Neurontin, Pfizer, lists as the recommended maintenance dose of Neurontin at 1800 milligrams, half of the 3600 to 4200 I was headed for.[1] They also state, "Dosages up to 2400 mg/day have been well tolerated in long-term clinical studies. Doses of 3600 mg/day have also been administered to a small number of patients for a relatively short duration, and have been well tolerated."[2] One thing I had no idea I was signing on for when he made this prescription was that it came with the possibility of thoughts about suicide or dying, attempts to commit suicide, new or worse depression, new or worse anxiety, feeling agitated or restless, panic attacks, insomnia, new or worse irritability, acting aggressive, being angry, or violent, acting on dangerous impulses, an extreme increase in activity and talking, other unusual changes in behavior or mood, since all of these were listed as possible side effects and I was headed for a dose far beyond what the manufacturer of the product recommended. If that meant I could possibly get to the point of overdose, the potential results were worse, including going into a coma.[3]

At the time, future medicine meant little to me. My failed operation was the dominant concern and I had all kinds of emotions. There was obvious great disappointment. I was also somewhat afraid. My hopes that this thing I carried inside me could be eliminated had been dashed and I was quite sure it would always be there, that eventually it was going to win. I felt like I had disappointed my family and friends and especially my wife. They were still stuck with me the way that I was. My hopes of not being a burden had made this all worth the chances involved, but I got the short straw. It was just going to be my life and who I was, how I lived, to be on edge about whether there is a safe place for having a seizure and always being tense when music was noticeable. Will my own daughter be afraid of me? The time away made me anxious to be back teaching school, as I was so lucky to be teaching the students I had, but it was nearly summer vacation.

We remained in Bethesda, Maryland, and I made a number of trips to Baltimore for appointments. An MRI was done, revealing that my right amygdala "had been removed." This small almond-shaped section, is paired with a matching section in the opposite hemisphere, like many parts of the brain. Together they control perceptions of such emotions as fear and anger while also controlling aggression. Research indicates the two on opposite sides do not duplicate functions, but have some specialization, which made my new lack of one somewhat of a concern. The right amygdala seems to be more engaged than the left one in retrieving emotional information and in a more shallow or basic general processing of information.[4] A study said that conditioned fear reactions or confrontation with traumatic events activated the right amygdala,[5] so not having one perhaps meant I did not experience those things the same as previously. My sister said the most noticeable change in my behavior following surgery was that I had "lost my filter" on conversation, and spoke more confrontationally.

Since I still had some problems with small seizures Dr. Lesser had me do 48-hour ambulatory monitoring not long after being released from recovery from surgery. This involved having electrodes attached to my head that were connected to a small device I wore which did a constant EEG to determine the location of the seizure activity. My head was wrapped with considerable soft cloth so no hospital stay was required. Friends Alice and Mike came from New York and we played bridge to pass the time. After several weeks, we then headed to Colorado, where our daughter was staying with my wife's sister. We took our daughter to a camp for a short stay and were headed to the mountain cabin where we usually spent summer vacations. On the way, we stopped in Boulder to shop. My wife was in a grocery store and I was in an adjacent sports store when I didn't feel right. That's the last memory I have until being in the Boulder emergency room, following multiple seizures. The Boulder emergency services contacted Dr. Lesser at Johns Hopkins. He thought I should return.

My wife and daughter remained in Colorado and I got a flight to Washington, D.C., then my sister took me to Baltimore and back for another week in the Epilepsy Monitoring Unit. All wired up again and with many crossword puzzle books from my sister, I was settled in. Dr. Vining was my attending doctor once again. Within a day of my getting settled in I noticed the girl who was occupying the room next to me. She was in the hall and appeared to be perhaps seven or eight. She was walking and swinging both of her arms. This sounds perfectly normal but the fact she was doing it is what made it so confusing. She was recovering from hemispherectomy and with my high school and college biology, I had learned how the right hemisphere of the brain controls the left side of the body and vice versa. Dr. Vining stopped into my room on her rounds. I told her I'd seen the girl and she couldn't do what she was doing. Dr. Vining just chuckled and said the brain is incredibly adaptable. She was a leading authority on hemispherectomies.[6]

Dr. Vining was involved in a study on following the progress of 54 children who had undergone hemispherectomies for incapacitating epilepsy at Johns Hopkins at the time and perhaps the girl in the next room was one of those included. I read about it the following year when the findings were released. I had spoken with her about this and seen her mentioned in articles, and noticed her in a *New York Times* story, "Removing Half of Brain Improves Young Epileptics' Lives."[7] Dr. Vining, who was lead author in the study that included other Johns Hopkins doctors, among them the neurosurgeon Dr. Benjamin Carson who would run for president many years later and became Secretary of Housing and Urban Development in the Trump administration.[8] Vining was quoted as saying, "We are awed by the apparent retention of memory and by the retention of the child's personality and sense of humor."[9] The children who underwent this procedure showed life with epilepsy at its most extreme. They were often having so many seizures that one episode pretty much blended into the next, and were frequently groggy from being on such high doses of powerful sedatives. While having the operation was clearly a desperate move, it proved to be a successful, life changing solution for some like the girl in the room next to me. The study Dr. Vining was involved in had speech transfer from the left side to the right in a 13-year-old boy, had found that memory is on both sides, and when half of the brain was removed, these children hadn't forgotten anything.[10] This certainly proved what she said about the brain being adaptable.

As for how the girl in the room next to me was able to be out in the hall using both sides of her body after removal of half of her brain, Dr. Vining's report offered an explanation, as reported in the *New York Times* article, "In many, however, strength and vision had already been compromised by the underlying disease, and the child actually became stronger after the operation rather than weaker."[11] Her brain had already been compensating for the failure and inefficiencies of the hemisphere that was removed, so perhaps without it she would be stronger.

I wondered about how my brain would recover from an operation to remove a piece of my right temporal lobe and related structure. Little did I know at the time that within three years a whole lobe and adjacent parts would be taken. Research says that memory declined after temporal lobe surgery, but this was affected by drug changes. With withdrawal from drugs memory might improve, but with introduction of new drugs it was likely to get worse.[12] A more recent study offered mixed messages that left me unsure. This found that "the data do not confirm concerns that patients undergoing temporal lobe epilepsy surgery are likely to develop accelerated memory decline over the longer term,"[13] which was reassuring. The same study also concluded, "Temporal lobe resected patients with persisting seizures however significantly lost within the long-term interval."[14] Since that was going to describe me, it was more disturbing, though memory problems could be attributed to many things, so it would be uncertain.

My stay in the monitoring unit was fairly uneventful until while watching a movie I had a severe seizure. One precaution for this is that in the unit they implant a heparin lock, a small tube directly inserted into a vein that is flushed out frequently and kept constantly open, so medicine can be quickly infused into the patient's bloodstream. For this 30-minute seizure, they had to make use of this and shoot Ativan, a brand of lorazepam which was a benzodiazepine, for calming the central nervous system.

Once I recovered from being sedated for this seizure event, I experienced strange auditory hallucinations that took different forms for several days. This began with me feeling like I could hear the conversations in the room next to me. Unlike my previous experience with auditory hallucinations these were not paranoid, just conversations between nurses about other patients, their duties, seemingly normal discussion. I also began hearing chimes at random times. This continued after my hearing other peoples' conversations ceased. I heard these chimes very infrequently for a couple more days even though I was released from the monitoring unit and the hospital. For a short time, I had a new experience, which was hearing my own voice coming from other places in a room even though I wasn't speaking. My brother-in-law and I stopped at a coffee shop soon after my release and I was looking over at the serving station often since I heard my voice coming from that area. I wasn't very interesting.

After several days of being out of the hospital that had completely vanished, but once again it gave me greater understanding of people who have their own reality and how it is not a simple matter of just telling them to get real and quit making things up. The sounds I heard during this time were as real as the sounds I hear any other time.

My wife came east when I was released and we stayed at my sister's place for a bit and went to see Dr. Lesser for followup appointments. I first did another ambulatory EEG for 48 hours with reduced medication where I could leave the hospital with my head wrapped and a machine attached to me got readings of all unusual brain waves. Then we returned and discussed how things were going. He said it was likely there was still epiloptogenic tissue remaining in parts of my remaining right temporal lobe but it would require more monitoring before we could consider further surgery to eliminate it. I didn't really know until then that more surgery was a possibility but I'd made my decision, trust the expert who does this every day and is respected internationally for what he does. He said more surgery so "we" were considering it. We also discussed the risks versus benefits a bit, a topic we would continue from then on in sort of a "cost-benefit analysis." While I had a great deal of confidence in Dr. Lesser it was my brain, I was the one who experienced the seizures, I was the one who was at risk when brain surgery was involved. We were scheduled to return to Singapore at the beginning of August. It was his advice that I not do so and remain in the States.

August came and we returned to Singapore and work. I soon heard from Dr. Lesser as he was going to be visiting our island from Johns Hopkins to meet with neurologists in the area who treat epilepsy. He was given fine accommodations and elegant meals were arranged for him with prominent people. Singapore was in the process of consolidating the government hospital services it offered into the National Neuroscience Institute at the time, so having him visit was appropriate. He had let me know he was coming and when he arrived it was his preference to avoid the formal dinners, as he wished to see some local sites and eat local food. My wife and I picked him up at his hotel and took him to Little India, driving down Serangoon Road past Hindu temples, then walked around a bit before stopping at an Indian restaurant we knew for a delicious meal. When we were walking back to find our car Lesser said, "The laws about driving must be different here in Singapore." I said something vague about not being really sure, but neither of my doctors had ever asked me whether I drove. Dr. Nei I-Ping had mentioned Singapore's laws once in a comment that included "draconian" and said there might be a ten-year waiting period of being seizure free at that time. Compared to most places that would have been incredibly long but apparently, it was more than that. According to the journal *Neurosciences*, Singapore was one of the countries in the world where if someone has had a seizure they can never drive.[15] I never asked since I didn't want an answer. That would change in coming years. While U.S. laws vary from state to state,[16] the Singapore requirement has become there is no set method for informing authorities of "unfit drivers," though there are expectations. The president of the Singapore Medical Association gave as an example of people who must be reported, "patients suffering from their first epileptic seizure or their first episode of severe psychosis."[17] There is that pairing of epilepsy and mental illness again.

I quietly asked Jane to drive before we reached the car. As we dropped Dr. Lesser off, he said he could show me slides of the procedure I would be undergoing, but I declined. The following night we picked him up again with my wife driving. This time we headed to the East Coast Seafood Center and had him try local favorites, chili crab and black pepper crab, caught the sea breeze and after dark, looked out at the lights of all the ships waiting to get into Singapore's busy port. My local doctor, Dr. Lim, joined us after completing his work, as he was anxious to meet Lesser. The two of them talked about conducting joint research and I suggested to Lim that he take Lesser to the Night Safari, a special attraction, then we parted. I would next see him in two months when it was back to Baltimore to have more of my brain removed.

14

The Grids

The school year began well and during "back to school night" I told parents that I would be away for a bit during the year. Beginning in October I would be at school on Sunday afternoons to hold practice sessions for a forensics event I coached, extemporaneous speaking. We held these long Sunday sessions since the event required students to give a seven-minute speech on any topic in current affairs with only a half hour preparation, so an important part of it was preparing detailed files on topics about news from all around the world as well as practicing giving effective and convincing responses to questions. It was November 1996 on a Sunday when we'd had a practice that I was driving back from the Singapore American School campus at Woodlands in the far north of the island. I was scheduled to be leaving for the United States and a longer stay at Johns Hopkins in early December. As I turned on to 6th Avenue, heading to our apartment in Pandan Valley, that feeling hit me. It was the tingling in my left hand and sense of panic that was familiar. I drove a bit farther then turned left off on a small road. After going only a short distance into what was a residential district, I turned into someone's driveway to get my car off of the road and pulled on the emergency brake, shut off the motor.

The next thing I knew was that my shirt had some wet spots on it, which indicated drool that often accompanies my seizures, but I was unaware of having one, or any time passing. I put the car in reverse and attempted to back out of the driveway but at first it didn't move because I had the handbrake on. Still groggy, I stepped on the gas and the car lurched to exit the driveway, since I hadn't released the emergency brake. As soon as I reached the road, I nicked a passing taxi. I then carried on to the nearby corner where unbeknownst to me there was a traffic cop on a motorcycle who was watching all of this as it took place. He turned on his flashing lights and pulled up beside me and I turned in at the next corner. The taxi driver had followed me and was there as well and I gave him my insurance information, though the damage was not of any consequence. The traffic cop was semi-polite but also convinced I was drunk. First, he asked whether I'd been drinking recently, then asked if I'd been drinking earlier at lunch. I said I was very tired, which was the case after seizures, and that I'd parked with my emergency brake on. He never asked whether I had any medical condition, but had me take a breathalyzer and said I would have to follow him to the police station if I failed. I agreed, and to his surprise the test didn't indicate any alcohol intake. He was quite frustrated, and said several times, "I know there's something wrong here." Very likely I was speaking with slurred words and the left side of my face was sagging, which was what happened to me after most seizures. A strange thing is that my words sound clearly enunciated to me at times like this, when I'm told by others that they are garbled or slurred. Since they exit my mouth and I have to hear them from outside, this is in some ways more confusing than when things are entirely internal. To the officer, I continued to insist it was just my extreme fatigue that was causing my problems.

I was aware enough to be very concerned about this somehow causing a problem that would require a court appearance, or do something that would prevent me from leaving the country as scheduled for my upcoming brain surgeries. To my good fortune a friend was driving by with her daughter, a student of mine, and saw me with the traffic cop. She stopped to inquire about the situation and offered to drive me home. The officer agreed that it would be a good idea and told me to go home and get some sleep.

That turned out to be a pivotal event. It was the end of my driving. I'd gotten my driver's license when I was 14 years old, the legal age in North Dakota where there used to be many boys who had to drive tractors and other farm machinery, so driving a car came along with it. I'd owned a car since I was 16 and been my wife's driving teacher before we were married and the principal driver since. But now, standing out, trying to convince a traffic officer that I was fine while feeling the unsteadiness that follows a seizure, it seemed like this was sort of a message. I shouldn't be driving. My idea that because I had an aura, it would give me time to get in a safe place if a seizure was coming on seemed vindicated, but that didn't make me very safe during the groggy recovery period. I would be most concerned about others, not myself, as the surgery supposedly had left a blank spot in my vision. Giving up driving in Singapore was not so difficult, since public transportation was available and convenient.

In all, it seemed logical, but emotionally was a different story. It really marked the loss of independence. A study done at the time I made this decision listed bans on driving as among the reasons people with epilepsy had higher levels of anxiety and depression than most others.[1] It pointed out that it wasn't the actual inability to drive as much as the underlying cause of bans on driving, and "the emotional sense of difference and inferiority which this may engender in the individual."[2] I suppose that was part of it, actually being more honest about the difference and inferiority. This made it harder to ignore. The "black blizzard" was taking a part of me now. As a more recent study reported by the National Institutes of Health observed, "Emotions triggered by driving discussions (especially by driving cessation) include sadness, powerlessness, frustration, decreased self-esteem, anger and anxiety."[3] Some of those ideas like powerlessness, frustration, decreased self-esteem certainly came with no longer being easily mobile, but that was what happened.

At the time, I couldn't really give it much thought because within a short time I was on my way back to Baltimore and Johns Hopkins. This was going to be different from when I returned for surgery seven months earlier. First, we went as a family. December arrived and we left the warmth of Singapore and made our way to Washington, then Bethesda. There was some time for preoperative work and orienting everyone for a stay of undetermined length, though hopefully we would be returning in something like a month. On December 3, I had an appointment at Johns Hopkins in Baltimore for a special MRI followed by a visit with a doctor from the neuroradiology department. He employed a technique that was designed to prepare special images that would correspond to an instrument he would use to direct his Wand. This would allow him to provide computerized guidance to Dr. Lenz, the surgeon, during the surgery coming soon and make it as precise as possible. It all sounded a bit like science fiction, but I assumed that was how things were now done.

There was a little free time during which we visited a friend, David Strauss, who was Vice President Al Gore's deputy chief of staff. He showed us around the vice president's West Wing office and we took turns being photographed standing where press conferences were given. My daughter, Anne, got the chance to visit the Oval Office. My sister made arrangements so she could attend the school that her daughter had recently graduated from, Holton Arms in Bethesda, Maryland. This is a private girls' school and she was going to be in small classes and hopefully meet some people. It would also be good for my wife to have Anne there with her so she could focus on her and not have all of her time being stuck with me in the hospital. Jane's sister also came to stay at this time, also making things much easier for my wife.

A second thing that made this visit different was that I was back for two surgeries, not one. The first was for the purpose of implanting electrodes directly on my brain to get more accurate EEG readings than the ones from the surface that pass through the skull and the dura so can be diffused. Dr. Lesser explained, "Implanted electrodes are useful when non-invasive methods don't sufficiently define what to resect in a patient, using them because they can record directly from the brain and therefore can help determine the site, sites, or regions of seizure onset with greater precision."[4] Once that operation was over, I would remain in the Monitoring Unit until there were readings from the implanted electrodes. Then there would be a second surgery to go back in and cut out tissue from the areas where the seizures were originating, if that was possible.

I discussed the procedure with my surgeon, Dr. Lenz, and my attending physician Dr. Lesser. They noted that my seizures had changed slightly since my operation the previous spring and I now had more focal jerking at the onset, but the right temporal lobe area remained the focus of onset. Whether that was accurate would be determined by what the implanted electrodes showed.

December 6 came, the day for the procedure, and I went into Johns Hopkins Hospital. The procedure seemed familiar. Again, a number of family and guests accompanied me and there was a small dressing room where I changed then waited. This time when the nurse came to take me down the corridor to the operating room, Jane and her sister, Judy, accompanied me briefly. They weren't allowed all the way, but we stopped briefly before I carried on. At that time, I said to Judy, "Take care of her." The question of whether I was going to survive the operation was once again a realistic concern. It would become more obsessive as I was rolled in my chair to the blue curtain by the operating theater again and was left waiting. The same chill gripped me as before as I sat there looking in at the surgical table and overhanging lights, alone with my thoughts.

Soon I was taken in and placed on the operating table, amid many people in the room. The anesthesiologist had inserted an IV and my head was clamped. That was the end as far as I could recall, except, once again, looking up at the lights and wondering whether this was how my life would end. Those lights will always represent that thought to me.

The operation was officially called a "craniotomy for implantation of grids, burr holes for implantation of strips." I was placed in the supine position with my head turned 45 degrees to the left side. It was then shaved, prepped and draped before Dr. Lenz began his work. He reopening the incision from the previous surgery along the question mark shaped scar that began above my hairline and extended to the bottom of my ear that he had used to remove a section of my temporal lobe and more from the previous May and removed the large bone flap. Following that he did crosscutting through the dura and took down the surrounding membrane to reach the brain. I was then given mannitol, a diuretic, which shrank the brain down considerably. Following that it was possible to insert electrodes on the surface of my brain. The electrodes came in pairs that were on strips of various sizes, with individual wires from each running to a larger cable. Once the patches containing the grids were placed on the surface of the brain Dr. Lenz would suture the patch in place. The largest patch of electrodes, referred to as Grid A, was a six by eight array that was placed on the back of the right side of my frontal lobe, all the way back to a fissure called the central sulcus that separates the frontal lobe from the parietal lobe. A group of 16 electrodes, labeled Grid B, was placed over the area where my previous temporal lobe removal had taken place and extended beyond. Strips containing 16 more were implanted nearer the back of my head in the temporalparietal-occipital cortex and called Grid C. Grid D was inserted on the brain above my right ear with four electrodes. A more challenging grid of eight electrodes was placed on the orbitofrontal cortex, located on the bottom of the frontal lobe. That was Grid E. Grid F also had eight electrodes, and was placed in front of E. The dura was then closed in watertight fashion. The bone flap was sutured in place and contacts for the electrodes from the grids were led through the skin before the incision was closed.

This left one remaining grid to be placed. To get access to the rear of the frontal lobe near Grid A required a special procedure. A burr hole, a hole that was drilled directly through the middle of the top of my skull, was necessary, and the dura was opened. At this point they encountered some difficulties. The operative report described what took place: "There was some brisk venous bleeding at this point which was controlled with bipolar cautery. We then made relaxing cuts anteriorly and posteriorly." A small grid of four electrodes titled Grid G was implanted, but "because of the granulations it was not possible to advance further or to place a larger electrode. The procedure was then terminated." Many years later I can still stick my finger in the top of my head through this hole, as well as burr holes on the right side of my head.

That was it and I had a total of 104 electrodes on my brain, each with a separate wire connected to an EEG recording device in a portable pack.

They wrapped my head very completely so I wouldn't mess with the wires and I was taken to intensive care for recovery. With that it was

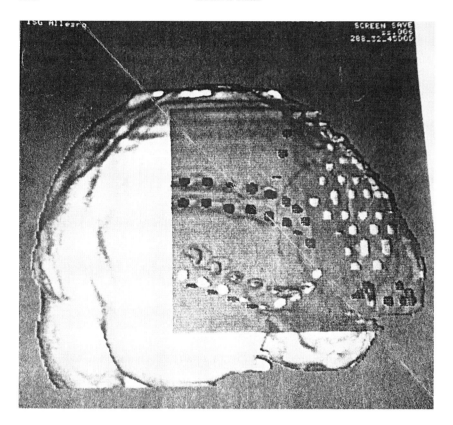

Electrodes on the surface of author's brain for more accurate monitoring.

possible for me to move, though there was an extensive, heavy amount of wire extending from my head which made me tense and also felt very strange. The doctors and staff were very concerned about brain infection, as bacteria can make their way into your brain by following the wires through the opened skull if care isn't taken, and hospitals are always swarming with bacteria. Meningitis was what they frequently mentioned, and with good reason. Bacterial meningitis can cause death within hours, and while most recover, permanent brain damage such as hearing loss or learning disability still may result.[5] Infections, including meningitis, have been noted in studies of children who underwent this operation, though they had their bone flap left off during monitoring that followed.[6] A more recent study done on a larger number of adults found 3 percent suffered from adverse complications including meningitis, though another study found it to be 7.9 percent.[7] The nurses wanted me to keep my head elevated a bit when I was resting in the recovery room to keep fluid from building up inside, though I had a drain.

After about a day I was moved to the Epilepsy Monitoring Unit where we waited to get results and find a more accurate focus for my continuing seizures. In the monitoring room my wife and sister were regular visitors. My wife's identical twin sister came and was there when Dr. Lesser stopped in while doing his rounds. He knew my wife well by this time but was taken aback by the sight of two of her. "I'm the backup wife," said Judy with a laugh, as she introduced herself. She had been doing a role previously that involved being responsible for our daughter, Anne. This time she was there and her husband Ron also made the trip. It was a relief for Jane to have their company as well as to be involved with Anne's schoolwork.

During my stay in the monitoring unit my room attracted considerable attention. I suspect a good share of the staff on the floor stopped in at some point to have a look. A box had arrived that contained the efforts of many students and was really a special treat. Two girls I knew well who were both outstanding volunteers at the leprosy home had somehow organized students to make 1000 origami paper cranes, many with personal messages written on them, and sent them to the United States from Singapore. This idea came from the children's book *Sadako and the Thousand Paper Cranes*,[8] about a Japanese legend that folding a thousand cranes would make a wish come true, and a survivor of the Hiroshima bomb who was dying tried to fold them. The author, Eleanor Coerr, had visited our elementary school and students on high school trips were among the many who brought strings of origami cranes to the Hiroshima Peace Memorial and hung them there. Now I had a thousand that were sometimes dumped on me, and another bottle of very small ones some Japanese students sent. Dr. Lenz, who was cutting into my head, found them fascinating and eventually asked me to find a copy of the book and inscribe it to him. I asked my daughter to make a string of ten for him, and she ended up making many for people. Years later after I hadn't been in contact with Dr. Lenz for some time, he sent me a note to say his son had read *Sadako and the Thousand Paper Cranes* in school. It was something special at a time when everything resonated more.

Early in my stay in the monitoring unit I was asked to sign a research form. I asked why and it was explained that they were using the opportunity presented by patients with electrodes on or implanted in their brains to attempt to do a more accurate mapping of where in the brain certain functions were controlled. Having all these electrodes implanted directly on the brains of people like me and others undergoing this procedure would provide a much better opportunity to do a detailed map of what areas in the brain control which functions of the body. A century earlier the functions of various areas of the brain could only be hinted at from clinical signs of disease or brain injury.

The most famous and informative case was that of Phineas Gage. In 1848 Gage was a 25-year-old foreman in Vermont for the Rutland and Burlington Railroad who was excavating rock. He drilled a hole and filled it partially with gunpowder. He was distracted and assumed one of the men working with him had added sand to the hole and commenced to tap it down with a 1.1 meter, 13-pound steel rod. There was no sand, and the rod caused a spark igniting the gunpowder, sending the rod directly through his head, entering below his left cheek and exiting the back of his skull. The iron rod carried on, smeared with brain, and Gage was thrown on his back. He remarkably regained consciousness soon after and was sitting in an ox cart writing in his work book when Dr. John M. Harlow, who had been summoned, arrived. Though Harlow cleaned the entry and exit points, Gage reassured him. Harlow noticed in subsequent visits that Gage had changed. Harlow wrote, "Intellectual manifestations feeble, being exceedingly capricious and childish, but with a will as indomitable as ever; is particularly obstinate; will not yield to restraint when it conflicts with his desires…. A child in his intellectual capacity and manifestations, he has the animal passions of a strong man…. His mind was radically changed, so decidedly that his friends and acquaintances said he was 'no longer Gage.'"[9] Gage attempted to return to work and travelled around New England seeking jobs. He displayed himself as a curiosity at Barnum's Circus, then returned to his family in San Francisco. He had developed epilepsy following the injury, and died in 1860 during an episode of status epilepticus. Lessons were learned from his experience. Dr. Harlow observed that his personality changes had been caused by the damage to the prefrontal cortex of his frontal lobes. Dr. Ferrier's studies on animals were demonstrating the same result.[10] Dr. Harlow asked the family to have the body exhumed so he could retrieve the skull, and it is now on display at the Harvard Medical School.[11]

This having my brain mapped entered me into a new area that has long interested neuroscientists, as they sought to construct an accurate homunculus, or "little man" that matched the cortex of the brain. This was first illustrated in 1937 by Penfield and Boldrey when they published a paper describing the result of stimulation on the cerebral cortex and used an artist to give a cartoonish rendering of both motor and sensory areas of the brain and what they stimulated. This was an attempt to display complex research graphically and simply. Thirteen years later Penfield and Rasmussen had this illustrated as cross sections of the brain with short bars connecting specific areas to the parts of a body sprawled across the perimeter.[12] These or later versions appear in most psychology textbooks.

Dr. Lesser didn't tell me at the time or when I asked him later anything about the specifics of the research form I had signed or what had become of it. I did see that years later he was lead author on a paper about subdural electrodes that discussed the relationship between stimulation and sensory responses. He concluded with "There is not a stable and standard representation of body parts, and an individual patient's functional representation will not necessarily match the classic homunculus."[13]

Though I wasn't aware of the homunculus relationship to the experiments I'd be involved with, there are other aspects

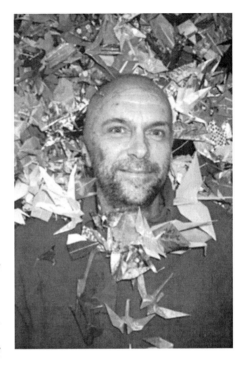

Surrounded by some of the Thousand Paper Cranes.

that interest me. The editors of the *Journal of Neurology, Neurosurgery & Psychiatry* thought that Penfield consciously chose the term and its derivation and that it was a peculiar choice.[14] It came from medieval alchemists who sought to change base metals into gold, and there were some who also sought to find a formula for creating a tiny person. This had moved beyond a science reference to modern psychology, which had adopted the concept of a little person with whom one converses in internal speech to provide explanation or interpretation for the outside world. A phenomenon which has likely become familiar to many.

I had very low current run into my brain according to my files. There was an extended testing time with an examiner that was designed to get more specific results. He and a couple associates sat in chairs while I sat on my bed and he asked me questions and gave me instructions. Usually while they did this, it just seemed like a good way to pass some time. There was one experience that was frustrating. I'd been asked something that I could answer easily and I was just talking away as though they were interested in my response. Not long after I began, right in the middle of speaking, the sides of my tongue just rolled up, and it seems like

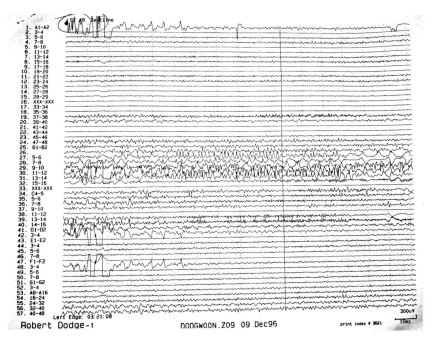

This and the following four pages show EEGs of seizure and corresponding electrodes implanted on the brain reacting. This determined areas to be removed in surgery.

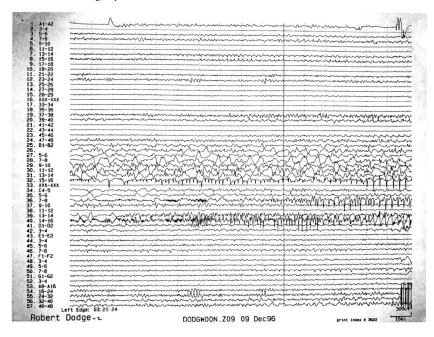

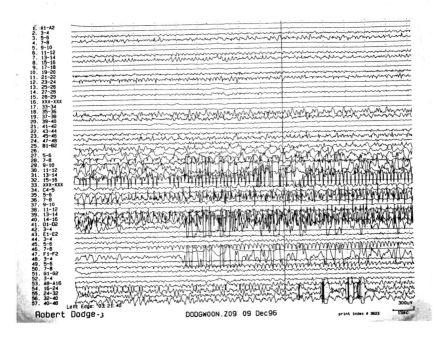

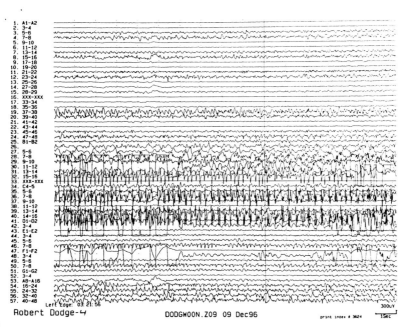

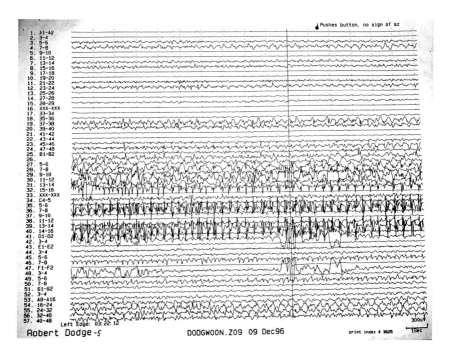

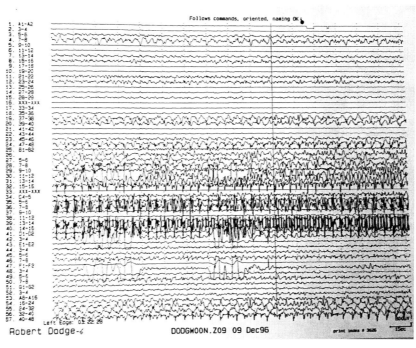

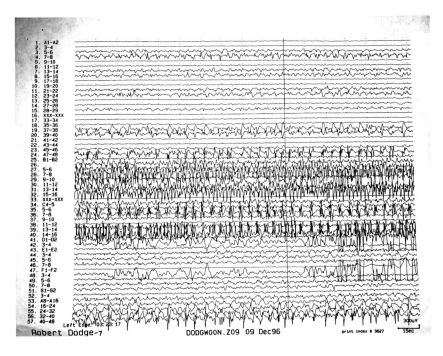

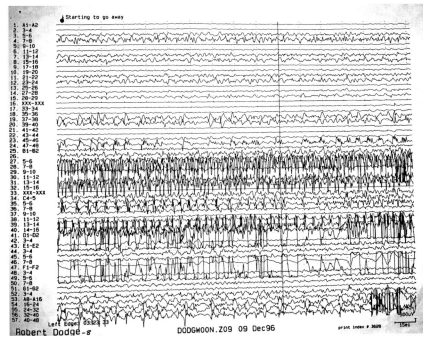

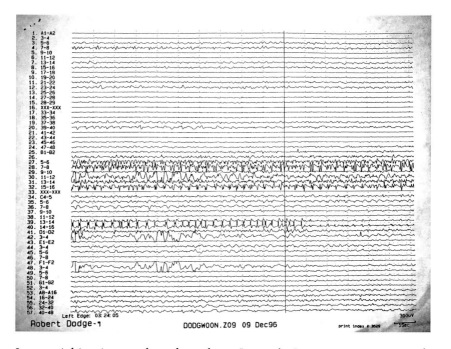

I was sticking it out, though perhaps I wasn't. In any case, my speech turned to total gibberish. The examiner who was conducting the experiment had definitely turned on the current for the electrode connected to the area in my brain that controlled my tongue. I found it really irritating that my mouth was doing things someone else was controlling, even though that was the point of the experiment they were doing. Apparently, this was all I noticed, as a report stated that "cortical stimulation mapping revealed sensorimotor representations for tongue and hand in the inferior portions of the A grid. No functional impairments were detected during stimulation of the anterior B and C grids or the posterior E and F strips." My hand must have twitched or something during the session, but I don't recall it being anything like the tongue. Maybe it was something normal.

Once I was in the Monitoring Unit I had five days of continuous video and EEG monitoring through December 11. The patient report was unlike others, since under the EEG section for each event it recorded the spiking sometimes by grid, but usually by the individual electrodes involved. That was certainly a more precise identification of location. Again, my medications were tapered off to induce more seizure activity, which was successful. In the five days, I had eight different events, "at least seven epileptic seizures," though they were generally mild as far as epilepsy and seizure go. They were simple partial and complex partial.

In the behavior described during these events, it was not as bizarre as my previous stay, but since they were mild I likely wouldn't have noticed some of them. While my behavior wasn't truly bizarre, it would have appeared strange to an outside observer, which again is disconcerting.

In the first two, which were simple partial, I could answer nurses' questions correctly, but in the third, which I had reported on the seizure button, there was confusion. While I first said that I was "OK," there was a doctor present and I couldn't repeat phrases for over a minute before recovering the ability to speak. That was soon followed by another where I could follow commands, but not repeat phrases and was shivering, but in less than two minutes I could speak correctly. A complex partial seizure saw me chewing, staring ahead, and unresponsive to nurses. Another that had aspects of simple and complex partial involved twitching, then jerking on the left side of my face and drooling out of the left side of my mouth, all within the space of less than a minute.

There was enough spiking recorded on the EEGs to better localize where my seizures were originating.

15

Third Time Lucky?

The MRI from my implanted grids was carefully analyzed by my epileptologist, Dr. Lesser, and my neurosurgeon, Dr. Lenz. Their critical findings were that my seizures showed sharp ictal spiking and activity arising from the right posterior temporal lobe and the right inferior frontal opercelum. It specified the electrodes to which this spiking corresponded. They also made what seems like a bold inference, considering it was more of my brain being removed that was involved, that didn't come as directly from the monitoring of the electrodes at this time. It did come from the fact that the seizure activity spread to the right inferior sensorimotor cortex and all of the areas bordered the superior temporal gyrus. When I had returned the previous June, and been in the monitoring unit and had the usual recordings done on my scalp, the temporal gyrus had been indicated as a site where seizures might begin. What's more, because I had auditory hallucinations at that time, or as my clinical report put it, "during some of his past seizures," they concluded that my superior temporal gyrus was part of my "epileptogenic zone." They could kind of pinpoint this, but would go for the areas around.

The map that was prepared for surgery now seems very primitive. So many things were being computerized by that time that it would seem like the guide for cutting out part of someone's brain might have been a computerized model after going through so much to find the specific spots that needed to be removed. What they had was a cartoonish outline sketch of the profile of a skull with a bit of brain, and someone had drawn little circles, or oblongs, 104 of them, where the electrodes had been placed on my brain. Each one was individually numbered by grid group, 1–48 for A and 1–4 for D. The grids were marked in recognizable, but informally written capital letters. At the top it said "planned resection" in poor cursive handwriting which had a red circle with an "x" in it as a key. Areas to be removed corresponded to where electrodes had been placed and were marked with an "x." The "motor" areas being removed, those that were related to control of movement, were noted by

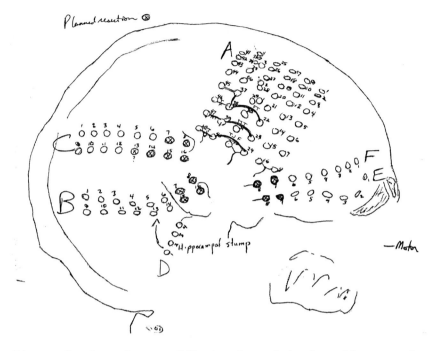

Diagram for planned surgery following electrode implants. Not reassuring for a complex and potentially dangerous procedure.

a red line over the circle that included the x. In all, it seemed like little to go on considering what they were doing, but it was a procedure Lenz had done many times.

They again explained the probability of the "pie in the sky" loss of vision that would likely occur in the upper left field of my vision. Far more disconcerting was a possibility they told my wife about, the chance of sensory agnosia, a loss of awareness that I even had a left side. This could mean when I shaved, I'd only shave on one side, I'd only brush half my teeth, I'd put on one sock and think I was dressed, eat the food one the left side of my plate and so on. Oliver Sachs wrote about this in his book *The Man Who Mistook His Wife for a Hat*. This condition is also known as "hemispatial neglect," and it occurs most often in people who have suffered strokes on the right side of their brain. Damage in the medial temporal lobe and hippocampus region, where my operation would be taking place, could lead to this outcome.[1] How strange this outcome could be. To live in a world where the left didn't exist was frighteningly described by *Scientific American* in a 2009 article, "Seeing the World in Half-View."[2] It described an articulate, intelligent woman named Sally who had a stroke and lost her left side, but was oblivious to it.

She used a wheelchair and bumped into objects on her left, ignored the left side of her plate when she ate. The authors asked her to touch her nose with her right finger which she did, then asked her to do it with her left finger. She paused and grabbed her left hand by her right and raised it to her nose. Things got stranger when they put her in front of a mirror so she would see her reflection and that it had two sides. They gave her a pen to write on a pad what she saw, but instead she lurched for the image in the mirror. When asked where the pen was, she said it was in the mirror. For Sally, left had ceased to exist, and in the words of the authors, "we should think of it instead as an existential extermination of the left side of the universe."[3] My wife was certainly concerned. She asked how to cope if things didn't go right and I turned out this way. They said she would need to put Post-its or some sort of reminder on the right side of things, so that I would know to look in another direction and find the remaining part or paired part. Even that wouldn't work in some situations, and this all really frightened Jane, as she wondered what life was going to be like hours from then.

On December 11 the operation took place. I was just moved from the Epilepsy Monitoring Unit to the operating theater. There is little in the records on the surgery other than it was conducted successfully. They just reopened the same brain flap again to expose the side of my brain and all those delicate parts were cut away, including more of the temporal lobe and small bits of the parietal and occipital lobes. The incision was stapled shut after the operation was complete and there was slight swelling and some drainage.

Of course, my head was considerably swollen and well wrapped when they took me back to recover. I wasn't kept long. During that time, we had some irritating news from Singapore. Apparently, there were people complaining about the cost of my medical care and how it would affect the rates they paid, since we were covered by a group policy for the Singapore American School faculty. It turns out I wasn't the only one who was undergoing expensive treatment, but there were people following reports of my progress, so perhaps it was more obvious. One problem during my healing was that my temperature reached 101 degrees. I really wanted to get out and felt ready. There were nurses taking my temperature along with other vital signs very frequently, including throughout the night. They would usually check my pulse and take my blood pressure then stick a thermometer in my mouth and say they'd be back shortly to check it. I got to a point where after they left, I'd take the thermometer out of my mouth for a bit and hold it by my face then stick it back in, hoping that would bring the number down enough so I'd appear fine and could be let out. Whether it was that or my temperature just soon returned to normal, I was taken off my IV and given a physical examination where my speech was considered normal, I succeeded on the finger to nose test for coordination that epilepsy patients so often take, my fine and gross motor movements were normal, and I could do the heel and toe walking, again a standard test. I still had the staples in my head that would have to stay for another week, but on December 15 they discharged me from the hospital. On the discharge document, they noted neuropathy and peptic ulcer disease. I'd been in nine days and had had two brain surgeries but it was over. The next question would be, was it worth it?

Even though I looked strange with the head full of staples, it was good being at my sister's home for Christmas with their family, our family, my wife's twin sister and her husband. During this time, our daughter Anne was invited to visit one of the girls she'd met at Holton Arms School that she had attended during my hospitalization. It was good she had the chance to get away from me and my challenges and be with someone her own age.

There are other things that became a little worrying, one not long after and some not until I read the hospital report. This was a fairly desperate attempt, involving two brain surgeries to really finally fix my problems with epilepsy, and what I had was commonly described as temporal lobe epilepsy. They had taken some of that lobe previously and did so again this time because it was where the EEGs showed my ictal spikes, which means my abnormal brain activity that leads to seizures, were coming from. There was also spiking in my right inferior frontal opercelum. That was something new, and more difficult. This spiking was located in the frontal lobe, the area where the high-level thinking functions take place and not where operations are easily done or even considered, unless circumstances are so difficult that it is worth risking the damage that could result.

When I first met Dr. Lesser and we talked about the possibility of surgery he assumed mine would be on the temporal lobe and I asked, "What does that do?" He said they really couldn't find any function, in that they were like kidneys, if you had one, you were fine. I never heard about the more detailed structures involved and just left it at that.

In January, it was time for me to check in at Johns Hopkins with my doctors so they could assess my progress on recovery. I was more optimistic than after the May operation, but not at all convinced. Things hadn't completely gone away. It had only been tingling in my hand. I'd been lying on my hand and could try to justify it and discount it because of that, but I recognized it immediately for what it was. The first time meant this all hadn't been a total success, and it had happened not long after my release from the hospital. I had the same experience again a couple weeks later, so absolutely it wasn't because of lying on my hand. While I hadn't had any seizures that involved convulsions or were really noticeable, the "black blizzards" were still there. Dr. Lesser had me reducing Lamictal and I was down to 400 milligrams daily by this time, while taking 4400 milligrams of Neurontin.

One thing he told me was "You have to recognize that you are handicapped." Wow. I'm handicapped, one of them. I suppose what was obvious to others should have been obvious to me, but I never really perceived myself as handicapped, even though I was well aware I had epilepsy and that it was a problem sometimes. But he was just telling me to be honest with myself and not be a denier. I could hope things were going to get better because of what they had done and maybe tingling hands were what it was going to be. If only.

I was to find out that this operation changed some things and took some things. It wasn't just part of my temporal lobe, which was like an extra kidney. It was my right operculum, which I would find out in an embarrassing situation. I'd grown up as a musician, had always been involved in music, and what does this strangely named section of the brain do? "The frontal operculum is sensitive to the processing of music-syntactic relations. Right frontal involvement has been observed for the processing of musical relations in melodies, mental imagery for songs, singing as well as rhythm and pitch discrimination tasks."[4]

So my ability to process musical relations in melodies for singing and my pitch discrimination had been removed without my awareness. It's not something you necessarily notice, and I was not informed that this was to be an outcome of this surgery. They didn't know I cared about music. I didn't really find out until Christmas vacation of the following year. We were back in Singapore and Christmas vacation was approaching. My mom still lived in Fargo, North Dakota, and we decided we would make the trip back to visit her. During my years growing up my dad had been the choir director of the First Methodist Church in Fargo and I sang in the choir from the time my voice changed. My favorite service of the year was just before Christmas, the candle and carol service. This was a special service of music and singing that ended with everyone lifting a lit candle. I thought it would be really special if we could get to Fargo in time to pick up my mom and for my daughter to have the experience of attending this service. It was really close, getting to the United States then making connections to Fargo. We arrived just in time to get to my mom and head straight to the church for the service. I knew all the carols and stood with the congregation, not holding back as I sang them out. It reminded me of years gone by. Jane was next to me and eventually she asked if I was aware what I sounded like, since I was nowhere near the melodies. That was a bit of a jolt, since I had no awareness that I could not sing in tune, which had come easily all my life. That ended any attempt at singing along with things or singing a few notes of the French National Anthem or something familiar while explaining something in history classes. Would I have objected or asked questions if I had been told about this before the operation?

16

What For?

In later January we were back in Singapore. Back to teaching, grading essays, normal life. There was something called Interim Semester at our school. It didn't really happen between semesters, but was intended to be an Asian experience for expatriates living there. It had changed over the years into a cultural or educational experience of some sort that took over a week out of the schedule early in the second semester, and in my earlier years, I had done such things as sailing in the South China Sea, trekking in Nepal, camel trekking in India, abseiling and caving in Australia. These trips cost extra money and there were some in-Singapore trips offered for those whose parents couldn't or wouldn't pay or the few who preferred to stay home and have a course that was over at the end of the school day. Having just returned from the hospital I wasn't going anywhere exotic or where my health would be the major concern, rather than me being the chaperone. I managed to join a friend, Andrea, who was doing a bus tour of different local cultural areas and sites, which was the right pace for me.

I'd had three brain surgeries and was taking a large amount of anticonvulsant medication but what had changed? About once every week or so I'd have a tingling in my hand that was now the main form my aura had taken. Apparently, the parts of the brain that had an effect on my auras being triggered by music had been removed. It seemed that way, though being nervous when music was loud had become such an automatic habit that it made me tense, even though it was looking like I might be safe with it.

Things went pretty well and in April we had spring break. We went to a small island Babi Basar, off the east coast of Malaysia. My good friend and colleague grew up in Singapore and he owned property on this land. When we first began going there it was secluded and a fishing boat would take us out, drop us in the water near the beach and agree to return several days later. By the mid–1990s there was a resort built and a dock so it was not quite the same. Still, it had a large two-story

134

longhouse, an open-air building on stilts with a thatched roof. There were cots that many of us took to the open second level where the sea breeze cooled the night. The main floor had some chairs and tables and the beach and sea were a short walk away, as were the toilets and showers. It was a place my wife and I and several other couples and their children had been visiting frequently ever since arriving in Singapore. That April I felt something go wrong when I had been wandering back to the longhouse, perhaps returning from the toilets, and I ended up in the jungle before getting oriented and thinking things were all right. I tripped over the edge of the longhouse as I entered and fell, hitting my head. I was clearly disoriented and whether it was the fall and hitting my head that made me so, or whether I fell because of a seizure and had not yet recovered from it is unclear. I apparently contacted Dr. Lesser about it because he wrote in a report, "Where they were on vacation he tripped over a hidden step coming in and fell, hitting his head. As a result of this he was somnambulant for a period of time."

The next month there was an episode where I remained alert but my hand began shaking. The school year soon ended and we were off to America and the Colorado Rocky Mountains. It was such a great contrast, spending the school year on the equator with palms and still some jungle around and summer vacation about 9000 feet above sea level overlooking Rocky Mountain National Park and miles of uninterrupted pine forest with Mount Meeker at just under 14,000 feet with snow running down from a crevice on the side, dominating the western view. After arriving this time, I had another experience where I felt tingling in my hand that turned to shaking. It continued as a partial complex seizure for four minutes and evolved into a tonic-clonic seizure for the first time since surgery, a real "black blizzard." Once that happened, it really started to become serious to me—what was it all for?

Following that we headed to Johns Hopkins for more evaluation, beginning with an MRI and EEG. My wife and I had discussions with Dr. Lenz and Dr. Lesser about my situation and options. Dr. Lenz took the opportunity to check on how my incision from the surgeries had healed and concluded my seizure was a result of the change in altitude. The discussion with Dr. Lesser covered a wide range of topics, including more surgery. We let him know that one concern in our decision would be insurance, as there was a limit on my policy and much of it had been spent on the Johns Hopkins procedures so far. He indicated that he would keep that in mind when making plans as for how to proceed. Lesser said that since I'd had the electrodes implanted it had become apparent that there was an area of potential eptileptogenicity, or one that was emitting irregular electrical activity, outside my temporal area.

He said it was above the Sylvian fissure in the rolandic area. The rolandic area is the motor area of the cerebral cortex and he thought they were not producing seizures, but only acting in concert with the areas in the temporal area that produced them. Lesser suggested it was possible my fall in April when I hit my head could have changed this and made that different, so it was now producing them. He wrote, "Given the risk to motor or sensory functions it did not seem indicated to remove that area then." There was an operation he discussed as a future possibility, should that area generate uncontrollable seizures in the future. It was a transection, which did not involve removing that part of the brain but instead, cutting numerous slices in it. The idea was that once a seizure began and started to spread, it would be interrupted upon hitting one of these slices and not generalize into a convulsive seizure. Then what about the conduction of the millions of messages that would also be interrupted by these slices? We never got to that point in the conversation, as carving up my frontal lobe seemed too risky when more pharmaceutical options remained available.

Looking at things before and after this makes sense, since the swelling from having encephalitis could have caused damage in several parts of my brain, making the removal of the one main focus mean there were still other parts that had been harmed. I'd had one status seizure and there were going to be more coming up. Having different active epilepsy centers in my head that could bounce things back and forth to keep a seizure going seemed logical.

Dr. Lesser also told me to gradually increase my Lamictal to 800 milligrams per day and cut Neurontin to 1600 milligrams daily. I had been nearly 3000 above this at 4400 milligrams of Neurontin per day coming into this appointment, where adverse effects listed by the manufacturer include such things as fatigue, dizziness, loss of control of body movements called ataxia, depression, to mention just a few.[1] These would still be high doses. Mayo Clinic has 500 as the usual top level for Lamotrigine, which is Lamictal,[2] and they say for Gabapentin, of which Neurontin is a brand, "the dose is usually not more than 2400 mg per day."[3] That's quite a bit below the 4400 I had been taking.

Again, I had been in a territory with drugs where I'm not sure of what the effect was on me other than being aware that I consumed more coffee than most people, and never really understood people who spoke of getting jittery from having a second cup. I was on a second pot before noon. It often made me think of the Robert Burns poem "To a Louse" that one of my high school English teachers had us read, and the lines "O wad some Power the giftie gie us/ To see oursels as ithers see us!"[4] Other than feeling a bit tired sometimes and occasionally having a bit of trouble with my balance, I thought I appeared completely normal. Looking at me from the outside during what were my often very high levels of sedative or other anticonvulsant medication might have presented a different impression.

In August we returned for the 1997–1998 school year. Not long after things began, I had a seizure after a prolonged aura that allowed me time to lie down and call for Jane. After she arrived, I pulled up to a sitting position, then the seizure came and lasted a few minutes. I recovered quite quickly, took an Ativan as a precaution against a followup episode. Soon after that I had an attack on a visit to Kuala Lumpur, then a tonic-clonic, or grand mal seizure that carried on for over 10 minutes, so this was not a good start to the year. In the first week of October there was another tonic-clonic seizure, lasting seven minutes and preceded by a four-minute aura where I was chewing and looking off into space. Through a fax exchange Dr. Lesser suggested that I up my dose of Lamictal from 700, which was as far as I had progressed, to 800 milligrams daily. I did, but things clearly were not under control. I tried going up to 850 on Lamictal, but found it affected my balance too much so rather than stumble around, I went back to 800. I also started on Topamax, which Dr. Lesser also suggested, but which was not yet approved in Singapore. Dr. Lim made me a part of the test group for the approval of the drug, with the added benefit of making it free at that point. Dr. Lim asked whether Lesser wanted me to stay on Lamictal now that I was adding Topamax.

Many students were aware of what I had been through and I took that opportunity to speak about epilepsy and my experience in a variety of classes. This included psychology, biology, health and I often included use of a video that had been a *60 Minutes* segment, "Martha Curtis' Story."[5] Coincidentally, this story on the popular news show had aired very shortly after I had been released for my brain surgery and it was about the same operation. It told the story of a professional violinist who had epilepsy and would have seizures while on stage. She had the same temporal lobectomy as I did, performed by a pioneer in the field, Hans Lüders, the man my Singapore doctor, Dr. Lim, had trained under at Cleveland Clinic. I had a copy of the tape made for Dr. Lim. It was good to have the chance to discuss epilepsy and the stigma attached to it with the students and I learned of a couple who also had it. I also was happy to be back visiting the residents at the leprosy home again.

During a class on Western civilization while I was sitting in front of the students in a comfortable chair, talking away and occasionally turning to write something on the whiteboard behind me, I had a tingling feeling. Usually when this happened, I headed for a nearby room, a teachers' area that was carpeted and private, and waited, got down if things continued and had a seizure out of sight on my own. This time it seemed like it would be all right, but it wasn't. I wasn't aware of anything until I was in a wheelchair, being taken to the nurse's office where there was a cot. Apparently, it had been a spectacular one. The assistant principal told me that students came to the office and when he arrived several were crying. I talked to them the next time we had class and many were very sympathetic, but it was the first time after all those years that I had a tonic-clonic seizure in front of a large group of students, a full class of them. What they thought, I don't know. Would they think differently about my daughter?

The seizures just kept coming, with two in February, another in March, one in May. Some were serious and I couldn't remember where I was after coming to, or couldn't respond to questions. These were the ones that involved convulsions, while there were others happening frequently that were simple partial and only caused a loss of awareness that passed, I hoped, unnoticed. It's more of the brain mystery that at times I would be lecturing and feel the tingle, know something was happening, but would continue. It sounded normal to me, though I know my words become slurred at times during these seizures. In most cases I managed to get to a private spot, but not always. Everything seemed normal and on a Sunday afternoon I was having a practice of my extemporaneous speaking team. This time it happened in a hall and only a few students were present, but students I taught repeatedly in A.P. classes and knew well. I wasn't only speaking about epilepsy, I was demonstrating it, which can be frightening to the observer and without information, can contribute to stereotypes and stigma.

Throughout the school year, I continued to make my regular visits to see the victims of leprosy at the SILRA Home. As always, it kept my condition and the stigma associated with it in perspective. There were always smiling faces waiting to greet us. Since there was no doubt I clearly had continuing problems, when the school year ended I made the trip of 12 time zones back to Johns Hopkins for more evaluation. That began with another eight days in the Epilepsy Monitoring Unit from June 24 to July 2. One thing I was aware of was a red patch of skin on my calf that seemed to have appeared and made me a bit nervous. Although the people I visited at SILRA had been cured, I interacted with them very physically and had shared food. I tried giving myself the test I'd been given by doctors in Singapore on other skin lesions or anomalies because of my time with leprosy victims. What this involved was taking a pin and not looking but slightly sticking yourself. People with leprosy have no feelings and will not be aware that the pin is sticking them.

What I had was a bit crusty and I expressed my concern. A doctor from the dermatology department who was South American came to see me, since he was familiar with leprosy cases, and examined my lesion. He said it was nothing to worry about and prescribed cortisone cream.

When I was discharged, I had an extended conference with Dr. Lesser. He said the EEG indicated that my seizures were beginning below, not above the Sylvian fissure so I would be a good candidate for further surgery to resect, or remove, more of the brain. He also said it would be best to do this as a process involving two surgeries again and do a grid implant first to better localize the site of seizure onset. After he instructed me to increase my Topamax to 600 milligrams per day and taper Lamictal to 300 our discussion carried on.

We talked about driving, which had become a matter of frustration to me by this time. I had said that because my seizures were preceded by auras that gave me at least a minute or more to get out of traffic and to safety that perhaps it would be reasonable for me to begin driving again. Lesser said that if that were really the case, then there were many jurisdictions where it was likely I could obtain a limited license with stipulations that I get out of traffic and pull off the road if there were any warning that a seizure might occur. I questioned him about the risks of repeated surgery, even though I knew the probability of it being fatal was quite small. What I was using is sometimes called the "gambler's fallacy," but I said if the probability of a fatal surgery was only 2 percent then repeating it four times, which I would if I did with the grids implanted, that would mean a probability of more like 10 percent. It's still really just 2 percent each time but one can look at statistics as one chooses.

Our discussion continued to the dangers of having epilepsy versus those of surgery and ending it. He spoke of two conditions that lead to death. One was status epilepticus, with which I was certainly familiar, having experienced it, discussed it with several doctors, and though I couldn't know it at the time, would be a serious challenge in the future. The other was sudden unexpected death in epilepsy, or SUDEP. I had heard of it but this was the first time any doctor had ever mentioned it to me. The Epilepsy Foundation describes SUDEP as "the death of a person when a person who is in their usual state of health dies suddenly and unexpectedly. When an autopsy is done no other cause of death can be found."[6] While it ranks second to stroke among neurological disorders as a cause of death,[7] the cause has not been determined with certainty and there is no known way to prevent it. The condition was first reported in *The Lancet* in 1868 when a British doctor described the phenomenon as "sudden death in a fit."[8] Much historical knowledge vanished since the early 20th century because most people with epilepsy lived in asylums or other institutions where staff had recognized that patients sometimes died during or after seizures. Our collective memory of these deaths faded as anti-epilepsy drugs became widely available and patients began living independently. A more recent example that supports this was a doctor who spent eight years in Tanzania treating epilepsy patients then left in 1971. She returned 20 years later and found that they had been without medication since her departure. She found that 164 of the over 200 she could locate records for had died, with half of those that she could find causes of death for being epilepsy, including status epilepticus, death during a seizure, or drowning or burning during a seizure.[9] Now most who die of SUDEP do so at home, unobserved.[10] The stories of suddenly discovered deceased children, wives, husbands are tragic and heartbreaking.[11]

In describing one of these tragic deaths, the *New York Times* added, "The extreme reticence of many neurologists to mention sudden unexpected death to epilepsy patients harks back to the days when doctors and families often did not tell people they had cancer—too terrifying."[12] Neurologists are "reticent" about mentioning this possibility to people with epilepsy. I imagine most would say that there is no reason to add anything else to fear for patients or parents of patients when they are diagnosed. A more generous view was offered by Jennifer Couzin in *Science*, who wrote that because of the stigma carried by epilepsy, "physicians swept SUDEP under the rug: They didn't want to magnify existing fears."[13] SUDEP is rare. About 1 in 1000 people with epilepsy die from it each year,[14] while the incidence in those undergoing surgical evaluation is 12 in 1000. Still, it is a real danger and there are precautions that can help, such as always taking medication on time, avoiding seizure triggers. In Britain, the national guidelines for 2004 recommended that physicians discuss SUDEP with everyone who has epilepsy, but a survey of British neurologists conducted two years later found "nobody told anybody anything."[15]

As far as what happens, nobody really understands. A study found that nearly all victims had regular tonic-clonic seizures, sometimes only two or three per year. A common belief is people they died from interrupted breathing, called apnea, or heartbeat, called asystole. Some researchers think it could result from the body's way of stopping seizures by unsettling vital brainstem functions and that breathing or heart failure could be the results, not the causes of SUDEP.[16] Anti-epileptic drugs have been suspected as a cause for SUDEP and two studies found that Carbamazepine, which is Tegretol, a drug I had been on throughout most of the 1980s, was an independent risk factor for it, though these have not been substantiated since. Another study found that patients taking three medications for epilepsy had a risk that was eight times higher than those on only one drug. Three is my current number and has usually been, though sometimes four.[17] I had a couple of the factors that showed up in victims, but no doubt that is true of many of the people with epilepsy, and it is more common with males having convulsions during sleep.

We discussed other surgical options available. One was the vagus nerve stimulator. This would be suggested to me several times as a less complicated procedure that has been helpful to people in a fair number of cases. I just wanted to get these things over with so my life didn't revolve around them.

17

Split-Brain?

To my surprise, Dr. Lesser also mentioned the possibility of me having a corpus callosum procedure as a treatment for the seizures that had continued since my surgery in December of 1996. A corpus callosum? When he said a corpus callosum he was referring to an operation that involved severing the corpus callosum, a corpus callostomy or commissurotomy. The operation is also known as "split-brain." It separates the brain's right hemisphere from the left hemisphere by severing of the corpus callosum, the swath of 200 million fibers that connects the two and allows cross communication between them. The purpose is for helping people with severe and debilitating intractable epilepsy, where seizures begin in one hemisphere and spread to the whole brain by passing to the other hemisphere through the corpus callosum.

Why he would even offer this as a suggestion to consider, I was unsure. Did he know things from the surgeries and the monitoring I had just completed that revealed issues that were more serious than I had been informed of? Had they thought that a more extreme approach was called for to prevent the situation from deteriorating seriously? In my current state this seemed like something a real expert like Dr. Lesser would not bring up without a reason. I was aware of the operation and had read articles about it previously in psychology classes and news and magazine stories. When the operation was in its early stages of use and the outcomes were being studied, the results were surprising. Headlines that followed those early studies included "Each of Our Heads Inhabited by Two Persons"[1] and "2-Brain Studies Hint We're 2 Personalities,"[2] among others. Those had caught my eye and had me reading about it even before I developed epilepsy. It was familiar enough that I had brought it up in classes I taught at times when conversations about the brain had come up. This was a really fascinating procedure. What I understood at the time, it was for controlling seizures in extreme, desperate cases and had implications not only for epilepsy, but also for physiology, psychology, and philosophy.

Cutting the corpus callosum as an attempt to deal with severe epilepsy cases had been done in the 1940s and "no significant behavioral or mental effects on these patients could be observed."[3] There was conjecture at the time in the English-speaking world that the structure had no real function except perhaps to "keep the hemispheres from sagging."[4] People commonly think of the brain as a single unit and home of the mind. With that mind, we have the ability to store knowledge and make decisions, think of alternative futures and make choices accordingly, to feel moral obligation, the feature that sets us apart from all other living creatures.[5] This operation demonstrated it was not so simple. It raised questions of whether the patients who underwent this surgery had one mind, two minds, or a mind that occasionally split in two.[6]

The formal study of the brain's two hemispheres had begun over a century earlier when a doctor from rural France presented a paper at a medical conference in 1836. He documented that in all of the 40 patients he had worked with who had lost their ability to speak, they had brain damage on the left side. Others confirmed his findings over time, while some noted that spatial perception was among the abilities damaged by injuries to the right side.[7] It wouldn't be until the early 1960s that things became clear and much more dramatic. W.J. was the 48-year-old pioneer patient with severe epilepsy who had undergone surgery to sever his corpus callosum in the laboratory of Roger Sperry at California Institute of Technology, or Caltech, in 1962. The immediate results were bizarre. "Seeing is believing,"[8] is how Sperry described watching W.J. attempt to match painted blocks on a simple pattern. He could do it with his left hand but not his right. At times his left hand would reach out and grab his inept right hand to guide it to the correct position. W.J. could easily name images presented on his right side, which were processed by the left hemisphere. However, he said he saw nothing when images were presented in his left visual field, processed by the right hemisphere. He could, though, use his left hand to point to a picture of the image he'd seen,[9] and manipulate objects with his left hand that was controlled by his right hemisphere.[10] The two hemispheres were functioning separately and each was capable of its own thinking. As Benedict Carey wrote later in the *New York Times*, "In a field defined by incremental, often arcane advances, the Caltech team had achieved a moon shot."[11]

Sperry and his colleagues, including Michael Gazzaniga, designed tests for split-brain patients to isolate the functions of each hemisphere, by allowing only one eye to view at a time, one ear to hear, one nostril to sniff, and so on. They did similar tests allowing both hemispheres to function simultaneously. They would flash a picture or show an object only to the right eye and the patient could report what it was verbally. When the same was done only to the left eye, the patient would report not seeing it. If asked to point to a picture of the object that had been displayed, though, the patient could do so accurately with his left hand.[12] In a similar experiment the word "hat" was flashed to the right side. Although the patient said he had not seen it, his left hand was able to locate a hat from a group of objects when the patient was told to select what he had seen. Then separate words were flashed to each side of a patient simultaneously and independently, such as "toothbrush" and "pencil." A collection of objects was placed before him and each hand reached in to find what it saw. If the right saw the pencil but found a toothbrush it ignored it, just as if the left saw a toothbrush and came across a pencil if did the same.[13] In another test they placed a concealed object in a patient's left hand that his right hemisphere could feel and asked him to guess what he was holding. The patient's "wrong guesses will elicit an annoyed frown"[14] since they came from the left, which could speak and hadn't received the message.

One experiment revealed a conflict between hemispheres. The patient was given a pipe in his left hand outside of his vision. He was instructed to write with his left hand what he was holding and laboriously made a letter "P," then an "I." He suddenly picked up the pace and changed the "I" he'd made to an "E," quickly completing the word as PENCIL. It is thought his left hemisphere had seen the first two letters and inferred the entire word. The right hemisphere immediately stepped in, took control of the hand and crossed out the letters ENCIL. The hand then proceeded to make a simple drawing of a pipe.[15]

What these and many more experiments made clear was that in split brain patients the left hemisphere housed language and verbal skills. The right hemisphere performed far better at tactile, visuospatial tasks, face recognition and line orientation.[16] In the popular imagination, the split-brain studies would eventually give rise to depictions of the right brain as the creative side and the left brain as the logical side.[17] This would become common usage and would affect education and other areas, though the ties to the science were tenuous. In the words of Michael Gazzaniga, "The language of these findings has become part of our culture: writers refer to themselves as left-brained, visual artists as right brained."[18] Those are descriptions, but as cognitive neuroscientist and historian of neuroscience Charles Gross of Princeton University says, "It became exaggerated and simplified to the point of being incorrect. It's true that certain cognitive activities tend to use one hemisphere over the other. For almost all cognitive activities, you need both."[19]

If the early split-brain patients definitely had two minds, then it would become problematical not to conclude on anatomical grounds that everyone has two minds, but we don't notice it except in these strange cases where they've been divided, because in a single body most pairs of minds operate perfectly parallel due to the constant and direct communication between the hemispheres.[20] As experiments continued and word of this got out, the reaction was curiosity and mystification. If people who underwent this operation appeared to have two separate minds after the connection was severed, didn't that mean we all had two minds as well? How are the hemispheres different? How would separate minds get along once they were no longer communicating constantly? Are we just one person? This conversation hasn't changed since.

Joseph Bogen provided an answer as one who had considerable experience with both corpus callosotomies, or split-brain operations, and hemispherectomies, the removal of an entire hemisphere like I'd seen at Johns Hopkins. His observation was that "the most striking features of the CCC [split-brain] syndrome do not and never have appeared in a hemispherectomised individual. The two-brain view is required to explain the CCC syndrome, even if such a view is not necessary or even relevant to other examples of simultaneous awareness and unawareness."[21] So people like the young girl I'd seen playing in the hall who was in the room next to me in the summer of 1996 at Johns Hopkins and had only half her brain left still had a complete brain according to this. She certainly appeared that way. Yet stroke victims often didn't.

In 1977 Roger Sperry, who had first demonstrated the separate functioning of the hemispheres on patient J.W. fifteen years earlier, gave an explanation of the state of knowledge at that time in a lecture at the Smithsonian in Washington.[22] He said that approximately 95 percent of the population have their main speech and language centers located in the left hemisphere. Following surgery, they saw no marked change in verbal I.Q. and "nothing to suggest that these are not essentially the same persons that they were before surgery with the same inner selves and personalities."[23] He then made it clear that in his view his research with split brain patients left them with two identities in one cranium saying, "Each hemisphere can be shown to experience its own private sensations, percepts, thoughts, and memories, which are inaccessible to awareness in the other hemisphere.... In this respect, each surgically disconnected hemisphere appears to have a mind of its own, each oblivious of, conscious events in the partner hemisphere."[24]

Next, he noted that some authorities have been reluctant to accept the conclusion that the mind is divided by the split brain, and maintain that it exists in the left hemisphere, the language hemisphere, or intact brain stem. They contend the right hemisphere functions only as a computer-like unconscious robot. "While these alternative interpretations may better conform with common concepts and traditions regarding the usual unity of the inner being, we have not been able to see any real justification in our test findings for denying consciousness to the disconnected hemisphere."[25] Sperry said his research showed the opposite, and over many years of testing, "clearly the right hemisphere perceives, thinks, learns, and remembers, all at a very human level."[26] He made correlation between what had been learned from the split-brain experiments and separate hemispheres with male-female differences, with females showing less lateralization, and discussed education and its traditional emphasis on linguistic training in the 3Rs and discrimination against the nonverbal, nonmathematical half of the brain, which has its own perceptual-mechanical-spatial mode of apprehension and reasoning, talents and abilities. Sperry also spoke of how this challenged traditional views of mind, self, person, adding, "It is no longer correct to think of a 'person' as being correlated one-to-one with a body, that we now need to sharpen and refine the concept in terms of critical brain states and neural systems involved."[27]

There was a lot that was mysterious but perhaps one result was the most frightening of all. This was the reports of split-brain patients who had two minds in their heads with different thoughts, memories, perceptions, that could result in problems when their hemispheres disagreed. Fighting could be taking place between two separate consciousnesses that existed in one head! *Science News* reported, "There is a case on record where a man's right brain took a severe dislike to his wife. His left hand was continually making obscene gestures at her and once tried to strangle her. Only by using his right hand to break the grip on his left could the man prevent an unfortunate result."[28] That person nearly committed murder in a struggle between his brain's hemispheres. Neurologist V.S. Ramachandran, director of the Center for Brain and Cognition at University of California at San Diego, told of a split-brain patient whose right hemisphere believed in God, but his left hemisphere was atheist.[29] How does that person act?

These stories point to the ethical issues that split-brain surgery has introduced. Sir John Eccles, winner of the 1963 Nobel Prize Medicine or Physiology, said, "These people come to us begging for help,"[30] but he raised concerns about the operation. He said it was "not in that class of psychosurgery ethically questioned because of doubts about whether the patients consented voluntarily."[31] This comment is interesting in that it raises questions about informed consent and patients' capabilities. In serious operations for there to be informed consent, how much responsibility belongs to the doctor rather than the patient? I've gone through a number of procedures where I am given a list of possible, probable, improbable outcomes before agreeing to the operation. In the case of this operation, it's the outcomes that are so unpredictable that giving consent really means your current situation is too difficult to live with, and if there are two of you, which one agreed? Dietrick E. Thomsen, author of "Split Brain & Free Will,"[32] acknowledged this when he wrote that people like him were not in a position to know whether it was better to live with this conflict going on within your skull or to suffer "high frequency grand mal epilepsy."[33]

Eccles also said that he would testify to an insanity plea for a split-brain person committing homicide with his left hand, which is controlled by his right brain.[34] The logic would be that with a split brain, the thinking and communication is in the left hemisphere and so this would not have been a rational decision unless the gun were operated by the right hand. While the author noted this would cover a very small group of possible defendants, he said drugs, psychic shock or other factors could produce a functional dissociation of the hemispheres, making this a less remote possibility.[35]

So right and left brains have "seeped into our vocabulary, if not our consciousness. We are already hearing the argument that functional disparity between hemispheres explains East-West differences, cultural diversities, artistic creativity, perceptual problems, and reading difficulties in children."[36] As for cultural differences, Daniel Robinson wryly observed in the *British Journal for the Philosophy of Science* that "the left hemisphere, like Western philosophy, is analytical, verbal, linear, and rational while the right, like Eastern thought, is intuitive, non-verbal, non-linear, a-rational. The inference, I suppose, is that Orientals tend to be left-handed."[37] Perhaps that illustrates the confusion between causation and correlation of the scholar he was referring to in his critique on split-brain capabilities.

So how much have we learned about the hemispheres, beyond that the left is commonly for language skills? Throughout the animal kingdom capacities are generally not lateralized. They tend to be found in both hemispheres to an equal degree. It is thought that in humans it could have been the development of language in a competition for cortical space that drove out the ability for perceptional groupings from the left hemisphere and that led to specialization of the hemispheres.[38] The right side is more emotional and "primitive" than the left.[39] Each half of the brain can control the upper muscles of both arms, but the right hemisphere can control only the left hand and the left hemisphere only the right hand.[40] There is a great deal of plasticity in the brain and some more primitive parts have been located where minimal communication between the hemispheres still occurs after the corpus callosum is severed.[41]

The interpretive mechanism of the left hemisphere is always constantly looking for order and reason, and creates it when it doesn't exist, to the point of inventing a potential past as opposed to a true one.[42] A *New York Times* story on this research said, "The left hemisphere takes what information it has and delivers a coherent tale to conscious awareness. It happens continually in daily life, and most everyone has caught himself or herself in the act—overhearing a fragment of gossip, for instance, and filling in the blanks with assumptions."[43] Dr. Gazzinaga, 30 years after being involved on the first split-brain surgery at Caltech, expanded on this role of the left hemisphere and language in constructing stories for the inner workings of the brain. He said, "Language is merely the press agent for these other variables of cognition. The mind may rule the self, but it is a constitutional monarch; presented with decisions already made elsewhere in the brain, it must try somehow to put on a good show of their adding up to some coordinated, sensible pattern. Functionally it resembles Ronald Reagan's presidency: It acts as if it were in control, and thinks it is in control, and believes it has good reasons for what it does, when in actuality it is often just mouthing soothing rationalizations while obeying the orders of unseen agencies offstage."[44]

Another difference between the hemispheres was demonstrated by Gazzinaga and a group of experimenters. They found that in people who had undergone a split-brain operation, their left side showed a bias for individual recognition, while their right side showed bias for recognition of a "familiar other." This experiment involved taking a photograph of a patient they called JW, as a reference to the original W.J. who had been a longtime patient of Mike Gazzinaga. They took a photo of Gazzinaga as well, then had nine computer-generated images that morphed together their faces, and transitioned them together at 10 percent increments from JW to Mike Gazzinaga. These photos were presented to JW scrambled in random order. The only question asked was "Is it me" or "Is it Mike?" and the 11 images were presented for six sessions to each hemisphere. His left hemisphere consistently tended to see himself in the pictures, while his right hemisphere saw Mike. This was repeated to see whether the results would be the same with celebrities rather than personal acquaintances. JW's face was morphed in the same manner with presidents Bill Clinton and George W. Bush. The results were the same, with the left side commonly seeing itself in the pictures and the right side seeing the familiar other.[45]

I had experienced the closest thing possible to split-brain when I had the Wada test, officially a sodium amobarbital angiography, where each hemisphere of my brain was temporarily anesthetized. It amounted to split-brain with only one hemisphere functioning at a time. In my case the report from the test showed no evidence of language or memory function on my right side, though I have a memory from my right side, one of frustration. Apparently whatever second brain I have is hidden pretty well. An experiment similar to the "Is it me or Is it Mike?" was done with patients taking the Wada test to analyze differences in the memories of the right and left hemispheres. In this case, they had patients memorize words and unfamiliar faces while their hemispheres were anesthetized. After their anesthesia had worn off the patients were given tests of their memory. What they recalled better from when they were under right hemisphere anesthesia and their left was functioning was the words. Their memory was better of the faces from when the left hemisphere was under anesthesia and their right was alert.[46]

While 98 percent of our actions such as heartbeat and breathing are automatic and not free willed,[47] there are other small differences between the hemispheres that are visible on the surface. The left side of the face displays more emotion. EEGs show that the right hemisphere is more active than the left when people are sad or depressed.[48] Patients with damaged right hemispheres are poor at comprehending sad pictures.[49] When people gaze to the far right and engage their left brains, they do better on verbal memory tasks. When they look far to the left, to engage the right brain, they feel more apathy and fatigue.[50]

So while I didn't know all the details, the split-brain operation was certainly familiar to me when on July 17, 1998, Dr. Lesser brought it up as a possibility for a treatment. His notes from our appointment say this doesn't "appear to be a particularly attractive option for the patient at this time." Not particularly attractive might be understatement.

18

Clearing Out the Rest

It was a new school year, 1998–1999, and I clearly had problems to deal with as far as epilepsy. Dr. Lesser indicated more surgery could be considered. One thing he suggested was that before having the resection, it would be useful to once again have a surgery to do grid implantation for more readings to find the exact areas that should be removed. He had mentioned the possibility of there being some irregularity in my parietal lobe. His recommendation was that Singapore was advanced enough in its neurosurgery at this time that I could make arrangements with my local doctor, Dr. Lim, to have the grids implanted in Singapore, then have the results sent to Johns Hopkins. He faxed a map of grid placement for me to give to Dr. Lim as instructions for surgery and mapping of points of epileptic activity. I replied that while I admired the Singapore General Hospital, it was my preference to not have brain surgery done by anyone other than Dr. Lenz.

Then there was another problem. I had reached the maximum of my lifetime payment on my health insurance policy, what with the cost of all the medicine over the years plus the appointments, then the visits to Johns Hopkins for stays in the Epilepsy Monitoring Unit, three brain surgeries, time in intensive care followed by recovery. I had a million Singapore dollar total lifetime policy and it was up. Now they were suggesting another surgery or surgeries, plus another stop in intensive care then time in recovery. But, if it is what Dr. Lesser recommended, it is what would happen, since I'd long since decided that he was the person I was going to trust. Jane and I had considered looking for new jobs while on vacation in 1995 in Budapest where we had good friends and several other former Singapore American School teachers had gone to work for a well-liked superintendent I'd met before when he'd been in Kuala Lumpur years earlier. I'd spoken with him and been honest about my health, but he thought he could get the school's insurance company to cover me. It seemed extremely unlikely, but with it as a possibility, I went to visit my superintendent.

While we didn't always get along regarding school policy, we could at least talk openly. I told him that because of the school's insurance plan, there was a chance we would need to leave the school and seek work elsewhere. We spoke about that for a bit and he said he would try to make an exception. He would present a proposal to the school board that the school pay all the expenses. It wouldn't be a precedent, since there were several people with serious medical conditions that were going to become expensive. The board agreed, which was generous, because it could be a six-figure amount.

I had a tonic-clonic seizure at work on November 9 that had been going on for at least 10 minutes when my wife arrived from the elementary wing of our campus to the high school. Singapore American School, where we worked, was the largest international school in the world and it now has 4000 students, but then numbered well over 3000 housed in a sprawling continuous building. The distance from where she worked to where I worked was considerable, though when she received word of my seizures, she knew the most direct route and was quick to make the trip. On this one, I was unresponsive and she feared it could continue to status, but eventually I regained enough control that I could be moved to the nurse's office, where I slept for two hours. The following day I increased Topamax to 700 milligrams per day. I also sent a fax to Dr. Lesser to inquire whether this was serious enough for me to consider a final surgery, mentioning that it seemed to have been suggested after my stay in the monitoring unit the previous summer, then things seemed to improve.

It seemed to be a pattern. When I started with a new medication the initial results were good, followed by a period of accommodation or something when the benefits faded. I mentioned that there were financial reasons involved in my question, since my employer had made me a special case and agreed to pay for what needed to be done, even though this had gone beyond what my policy would pay. I added that this benefit could be temporary, and might not exist in another year. I added that while this was not a reason for having surgery, it was something I needed to consider. Additionally, I asked him when surgery might be a possibility, mentioning that I'd thought of Christmas. No doubt that was too soon and it would be essential to me that it happen when he and Dr. Lenz were both available. I suggested perhaps June or July.

Lesser replied the next day, saying Dr. Lenz was away and he'd discuss it with him when he returned. He replied later in the month, saying there were two options: further removal of the temporal lobe and putting in a grid above the Sylvian fissure, meaning in the frontal lobe, where the appropriate procedure might be a multiple subpial transection. Research showed the latter operation had reduced patients' word fluency and could also impair both their motor and language abilities.[1] I really wasn't very interested in having someone cut slices in my frontal lobe, though it might have been helpful for what was going to come later as my seizures became more severe.

In January of the new year I sent a fax to Dr. Lenz, my surgeon, and said that the seizure activity in the posterior frontal lobe I had that was indicated by the EEG from the grid implant he had done was not found on my stay in the monitoring unit during the past June. Additionally, I was not interested in a second grid to determine the precise location of focal point or points that remain, and in weighing the risks of a transection against the possibilities of success and the amount of improvement it would bring to my life, it didn't seem like a difficult choice. Though I'd recently had another serious seizure, my life was not interfered with to a great degree. I said our school year ended on June 4 but I would make myself available to work around his and Dr. Lesser's schedules, since their presence was essential, and would come at any time from that point on.

They contacted me in April and said that there would be an available time at the beginning of June. I couldn't finish the school year, but got through AP exams and headed back to the United States again a bit past mid–May. I met with Dr. Lesser and discussed the procedure with my sister present. He said the stump of my temporal lobe would be taken, so it would be entirely removed and the occipital lobe would also be touched. There would be more. My wife and daughter Anne finished the school year and then they joined me. It was all pretty familiar now and I had appointments, got prepared mentally and physically. We had a little family time, then I was in the hospital for brain surgery number four.

It was June 6 and once again I changed into a gown in a small room before waiting to be picked up by someone to transport me to the operating theater. Whether it was a nurse or an orderly I don't recall, but the experience was the same. It was that quiet ride in a wheelchair, then being left alone where I could peek in an opening in the blue curtain and see the operating table sitting there, waiting for me under large lights. All the same feelings as before about whether this was it, and whether I would not be getting through this one. By this time, I'd kind of given up on optimistic thoughts about how this might be the time it was going to work, that I'd be coming out of this great and when I woke up epilepsy would just be a memory. I think I was fairly resigned to my fate that it was just part of who I am. Again, I looked up at the light as the anesthesia was administered and tried to count back from ten, hoping that I would wake up again.

When I passed out my head was shaved and prepped then the old question mark shaped incision on the right side of my skull was opened for the fourth time, using a drill to follow the previous incisions. Once this was finished the bone flap on the side of my head was elevated but when they did this, the brain stuck to the back edge of the dura from the previous operation. Once this was separated and they had a clean dural edge they worked along the previous incision to the lateral wall of the Sylvian fissure that separated the lobes. They identified the different regions and moved to the previous resection, then took what remained of the temporal lobe and also the remainder of the hippocampus. Some tissue thought to be hippocampus on the MRI scans turned out to be scar tissue. They cauterized the areas that had been cut. Perhaps there was some blood pressure problem, as the operative report says, "The patient had a Vasalva before closing," in a reference to a maneuver that is sometimes used to reduce high blood pressure. Following that, the dura was closed with nylon stiches and a mesh inserted, the bone flap was replaced and the skin stapled closed. Titanium plates with bolts held the skull together, but an epidural drain remained to allow the blood and excess fluid to clear from the operation.

Before long I was out of recovery and back in a room. Missing an eighth of my brain is what a recent epileptologist of mine told me. Of course, I was swollen and uncomfortable. One afternoon soon after while I was alone, a woman entered the room who really took me by surprise. I didn't recognize her at first because she was so out of place. She was the mother of a student I had in Singapore, a wonderful girl, Alice, who had Marfan syndrome, a condition that causes people to become unusually tall and thin. Alice had come for surgery on her back to see if that would help. Her mom hadn't been impressed with the Johns Hopkins food service and had found a Chinese restaurant she thought was satisfactory. That night she brought me small boxes of Chinese food, as she thought I must be missing it.

When I had a couple days to rest, my wife had thought it was time for Anne, our daughter, to see what I was going through, and she brought her to the hospital to visit. By this time, she was 14 and had seen me have seizures, but this was different. There I was with my big swollen head with the question mark of staples and yuck running out from my brain. And she was going to be in high school in the fall, so we'd be seeing each other in a different setting soon, but she'd always have this vision of me. My brother and his wife flew from Berkeley to be there as well. My sister had suggested it, as she had seen me in all the operations and thought my brother should know what I'd experienced. Bob, a very close friend from high school, also came by, so the recovery time passed.

Upon being discharged the nurses undid the tubes I'd been attached to and had me sign a form, then let me go. One of the tubes was a heplock, which I was always on whenever in the hospital. It was a short tube to keep a vein open in case I happened to have a seizure that turned to a status seizure and they needed to be able to administer some serious anticonvulsant medication while I was having continuous violent seizures. Jane and I walked to the elevator in the Meyer Building where all the neurology work was done at Johns Hopkins, and headed down from the fifth floor to the main level. On the way, the small Band-Aid that was covering the site of my heplock was soaked, then soon there was much blood rushing from my arm to my shirt, also staining a wide leather belt I was fond of. We went back to the checkout counter for a second try, and they put on gauze and tape while apologizing, then we made a second attempt and found our way to the parking lot.

As for this surgery being the answer, once again it wasn't. There was no hopeful period. Dr. Lesser's notes say I had several seizures in the immediate post-op period followed by periods of panic, while Dr. Lenz's say I had one. Lesser wrote that the symptoms could clear in a month or two, "Time will tell." They both mention that I was having vision problems, with Lenz commenting on an upper left quadrant defect, while Lesser wrote of how I had changes in my vision and often felt like I'd just been looking in a bright light which caused everything to become darker. He said the numbness in my feet seemed to have increased as well, and suggested I get some sort of medical alert bracelet or necklace. Since I was released and it was summer vacation, we were heading for Colorado and the mountains, but he said I should rest at high altitudes.

Dr. Lenz told me to go and "enjoy the cranes," remembering the paper cranes from the previous operation and he still had the string of ten my

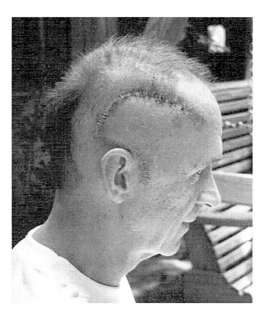

Awaiting having my nephew remove my staples after being released from hospital.

daughter had made hanging from the corner of a frame in his office. I really appreciated his advice. He said some patients become more than patients, they become friends, and he hoped I'd be able to enjoy what I had. It was a thoughtful gesture that I appreciated, and while I know both he and Dr. Lesser and all the other very highly trained, very skilled and expert people at Johns Hopkins had done what they could, the future wasn't going to get brighter soon.

19

Carrying On

After a summer in Colorado we were back in Singapore for another school year. I continued doing the things that I'd done in the past, taught the same courses and regularly visited the leprosy home, coached the extemporaneous speaking team, got together with friends. I was pretending the surgeries had been successful, but was still having auras, so things were still happening in my head. This fantasy didn't last long. While I'd remain fully conscious, I began having simple partial seizures at times and complex partial seizures about every other month. When they happened, I usually just didn't speak or look around and tried to get through the episode without being noticed, and often got away with it since they were brief. That was easiest when they were simple partial, and if I just kept to myself there was little to notice. There were times they weren't as mild, the complex partial seizures, when I knew something had really happened. These were limited and only affecting small areas of my brain, though they made me very nervous and unsteady. With those I sometimes drooled slightly and I'd feel totally aware and my hearing remained fine. If I had to speak during these, it sounded accurate to me, though to others, it was likely somewhat slurred. Jane could see it in the left side of my face when either was happening, and a couple of others would ask if I was all right. I would nod yes, as I didn't want to speak.

My awareness meant the seizures were being confined to one side at most. That was true until it wasn't. In that fall at school I escaped to a secluded area and had a tonic-clonic seizure. Several months later I was at home on our ground floor near the entrance to our house and felt something coming on. I moved to the narrow couch in our living room beneath the ceiling fan and lay down to be prepared. Then came another very violent seizure which had Jane and our maid standing beside me and blocking me as I convulsed, trying to keep me on the couch to prevent me from falling on the marble floor. Having these generalized seizures really was a setback. Four brain surgeries and all this medicine and I was having the very problems that started everything over 20 years earlier. But there were no options other than carrying on and seeing what came next.

I visited Dr. Lesser a year after my operation and had an extended EEG of about two hours where they hoped I'd sleep among other things. The tests showed spikes in the frontal temporal lobe and also a spike in the posterior frontal lobe. The conclusion from this was "This combination of findings suggests that further resection would not necessarily stop his seizures, at least if the resection was done in a simple way. For this reason, we should continue to concentrate on medications." I guess that was good. No more going through the surgery and keeping the remainder of the brain that I had. And the line you always hear is that there are new medications being developed. There were some being used with success that I hadn't tried.

Following that I remained at my sister's home in Bethesda, Maryland. My former professor, Thomas Schelling, now lived there as he had taken a job at the University of Maryland since his age required retirement and had an office near my sister's. We had kept up correspondence over the years about my teaching his work on game theory to high school students. We had gotten together after my last surgery and when speaking informally I'd said he should be writing his memoirs, since he had been the foremost civilian advisor on nuclear strategy during the Cold War and had been involved with presidential administrations from Truman through Nixon. He said he wasn't interested in spending the time and I had volunteered that I would certainly be willing. The result was that in the summer of 2000 I spent eight days in June at his home taping him and getting his recollections and would return from Colorado again in July for another session as well as the more later. Interspersed with that was an appointment with Dr. Lesser, who said "the patient thinks that Topamax has helped him more than Lamictal." I recall that conversation and him asking me which of the two medicines was more helpful and my saying that there was no possible way I could tell. He told me that I could. At that time, I was taking 600 milligrams of Lamictal and 700 milligrams of Topamax daily, both doses above the highest level recommended by the Mayo Clinic,[1] which resulted in regular drowsiness.

When I began my interviews with Schelling initially, I'd take an Ativan as a preventative measure before these meetings as they were events where a seizure of any sort would have been more than a distraction. This was an honor, to spend so much time with this great man and his wonderful wife, Alice, and hear the history that he had at his fingertips and his being involved in events where the world's fate was at stake. It gave me a new focus and sense of purpose. In time, it would give me some pride and a bit of dignity, something it's easy to lose when you have epilepsy. That was about to become more obvious.

Once we were back in Singapore, I was up to 700 milligrams of Lamictal and 700 milligrams of Topamax daily but my problems were still present. I had a mix of seizures, including simple partial where I retained awareness and complex partial where sometimes I didn't. Also, there was another tonic-clonic seizure. One especially frustrating day came when my wife and I were downtown walking along Orchard Road, Singapore's best-known street and the heart of the shopping district. It's always interesting because there is so much happening even if we just wanted to wander around and stop for lunch or coffee and not shop because the city is so cosmopolitan and there are so many tourists from East and West that the people watching was always fun. On this day, I turned out to be the object of attention. We happened to be in front of Ngee Ann City, also called Takashimaya, which is one of the largest shopping centers in the city and has an enormous entryway with a gradual staircase. I didn't feel well and it turned out it was a seizure coming. I got down on the sidewalk and waited, then it happened. It was short, but I was very disoriented and not coming out of it, so I just remained there on the crowded sidewalk. Jane recalls that no Singaporeans offered to help, though there would have been thousands passing. Several Europeans asked if there was anything they could do, but she said I just needed some time to recover. Eventually a guard from Takashimaya, the shopping center, came over and asked Jane to move me because I was scaring away customers by lying there in front of their entrance on the sidewalk. Jane told him she would when I was ready to move. He didn't push it anymore. I was alert enough to be aware enough of the conversation but not to participate. It was, of course, humiliating to be a public nuisance in front of a crowd of people. Most of them probably thought I was drunk and couldn't walk, so their lack of sympathy was perhaps somewhat understandable. I know it's a feeling others with epilepsy can identify with following a public seizure—embarrassment, compounding the feelings of irritation and helplessness when lying there unable to do anything about it on your own. So often I had Jane to help, but not always.

Lesser's nurse contacted me to say she had discussed the possibility of my having Diazepam Intensol available for emergency situations. I continued to use Ativan and would get a prescription for Diazepam at my appointment with Dr. Lesser when I returned to the United States at the end of that school year in 2001. There was a major advantage of Diazepam. It was a liquid and was absorbed through the mucous membrane, so if administered in the cheek or under the tongue it was absorbed directly into the bloodstream. It didn't need to work its way through the digestive system so it was in one's body more quickly than other emergency medicines a person could have in his possession. Because of this, it is also a drug of first choice for treatment of early status epilepticus and acute repetitive seizures.[2] It turned out to be inconvenient, as it came in tubes that were designed to be inserted in a syringe and injected into a patient by first responders. My nephew Dave, an emergency room doctor, used a syringe to transfer all the medicine to small tubes that could be opened. Additionally, there had to be an eye dropper kept with them to measure out 5 or 10 milligram doses to be squeezed into my mouth. It needed to be refrigerated so I kept most at home and a small supply in a mini-fridge in my classroom. Our maid in Singapore learned the amount to administer by eyedropper and the time would come when I began having a seizure on our couch and she did the procedure correctly. I don't know whether it was the medicine, but the seizure did not last long and I didn't end up in the hospital.

I didn't have it available at the time it might have helped shortly after seeing Lesser. Our summer routine was to spend time at my sister and her husband's cabin in Colorado not far from Estes Park. Then before heading back we went to Aspen, where again we welcomed their generosity for a week stay, then made the great change in latitude to Singapore. My brother-in-law taught at the Armed Forces Institute of Pathology and regularly ran a medical conference in Aspen in late July, early August and for years, invited us to spend one of the weeks there, which came during the Music Festival so there was lots of activity. We were staying at the very pleasant Ritz-Carlton Hotel, and Jane and I were among others who settled in a hot tub to enjoy the evening as it cooled down. I started to feel bad and got on the side but soon I shocked everyone and was having a full-blown seizure. It stopped, then started again, but I had briefly regained a glimmer of awareness between the two. The second seizure stopped but was soon followed by another and Aspen emergency services were called. Not surprisingly Aspen has good emergency health care services and they soon arrived and ripped pads from chairs to protect my head. Even though I was convulsing violently they managed to get a needle in a vein somehow as I flailed and get me to a clinic. It had seemed like status because it carried on for so long, but it wasn't. Their diagnosis on my report was "multiple seizures," which are now commonly referred to as "cluster seizures." This was really the "black blizzard" lurking in my head announcing all the procedures and medicine hadn't eliminated it, and it could burst through to overwhelm everything, and saying eventually it was going to win. A study reported in *Epilepsia* found that there is a correlation between cluster seizures and convulsive status epilepticus, telling physicians to be aware of this danger with patients they treat.[3]

In an impressive display when a van from the hotel brought me back the following day, the entire staff was standing outside to greet me and I was given flowers. Every employee sent a card to our room. It was surprising and totally unexpectedly friendly and welcoming.

We headed back and the situation persisted. I had my mix of different kinds of seizures. There was another humiliating time when spring break came. The three of us, Jane, Anne and I, went to Paris to stay on the left bank in a hotel that had been an abbey in the Saint Germain area and had been converted into a boutique hotel. It was Anne's first exposure to Paris and the culture centered there as well as the food. We usually walked or traveled by Metro and Jane and I had many fond memories of the city that we hoped Anne would also enjoy. One evening we were taking a walk down Boulevard Saint-Michel in the Latin Quarter and I had an aura that persisted. When it lasted too long, I got down on the pavement, trying to get out of the flow of walkers and near a building. After first sitting, I thought I should lie on my side, and I had a brief seizure. Like in Singapore, I was ignored by those passing by. I hadn't convulsed or done anything dramatic and while it was soon over, I was groggy from the experience. It could well be that people assumed I was drunk and had no sympathy or thought of offering help, though there I was, this time with both my wife and daughter present, lying on the concrete as people went by, with more disdain than sympathy. Another attack on my self-respect, not for choices I'd made but for having a condition over which I seemed to have little control. Those "black blizzards" buried in my head struck again, even if not violently, it was still another chip at struggling to have self-respect as I lost it from others.

Our trip finished and we returned, but I wasn't done disrupting my daughter's life. As for others with my condition it was especially deflating when it imposed on the lives of those closest to me. I was fine the day my students had their Advanced Placement exams but on the morning my daughter was to go in for her AP Biology exam I had a tonic-clonic seizure, clearly a very upsetting experience for her. Arrangements were made and she was able to take her test, but my life was imposing itself on hers at an unfortunate time. The following year was her senior year and she had done very well in high school, academically, socially and in activities, most noticeably dance but also others.

I had an increase in dramatic convulsive seizures that year, including one on our block on the opposite side of the park in front of our home, where after heading down to the nearby trail by the canal for my exercise walk in the heat of the day, I was returning but ended lying in someone's driveway and a small crowd gathered. Our home was an attached condo that we rented and some were detached houses, but all surrounded a small park and had Filipino maids who worked for far too little and in some cases, had very little free time. But after finishing chores at night they often gathered in the park and spoke in Tagalog and occasionally had Philippine food together. They had a regional communication network where word spread quickly. The residents of the home where I had my seizure were about to call an ambulance when word arrived at our house through the maid rapid communication system. Our maid told our daughter who was there within a minute, and by that time the seizure had ended. Like her mother, she took charge and instructed them not to call an ambulance since there was no emergency, it was just what happens and then it was over. These were Chinese neighbors as were nearly all in our neighborhood and this young Chinese woman who spoke English had told them what to do with this middle-aged white man. All the maids knew the situation and we'd lived in the neighborhood long enough that most people had likely seen us and were polite, though they didn't really welcome us.

That was one of four tonic-clonic, or grand mal seizures that year but there were others as well, even though I'd gone up to 900 milligrams of Lamictal while remaining at 700 of Topamax. By then the Lamictal was far beyond the recommended maximum and Lesser said that doses above 700 of Topamax had not shown to be any more effective. Dr. Lim, my Singapore doctor, generally deferred to Dr. Lesser since I'd exchange emails with Lesser before my Singapore appointments to ask for his suggestions on what to try next as well as seeing him during the summers. Dr. Lim suggested following one of my seizures that I consider a vagus nerve stimulator. Lesser had mentioned it previously as a possibility as well. I said it didn't seem appropriate for me, but was more for someone who had very frequent seizures and he agreed. I also contacted Dr. Lesser for his opinion, and he wrote a thorough reply. He said it could be a help but not a cure, adding, "About a third to forty percent of patients have a fifty percent or greater reduction in seizures." Those could be odds worth risking. He described what was involved: "The stimulator is a device that is put in the chest, something like a pacemaker. It connects to a nerve in the neck, the vagus nerve. By mechanisms that are unknown, stimulating the vagus nerve seems to reduce seizures in some people. There is also laboratory evidence supporting this so it's a real effect. The problem is it doesn't seem to control seizures completely and doesn't always work. The major side effect is that when it stimulates the vagus nerve you get a tickling sensation in the throat." He said I'd have to come and stay a few months to get the stimulator computer program properly adjusted unless it could be done in Singapore. He added, "The other option is to wait for new medications or new approaches to problems like yours." I wasn't interested in another operation right then and I knew we were talking about other medicines.

20

Heavy Weather—
"Black Blizzards" Strike

Our daughter graduated from high school in 2003 and headed to the United States for college. Though we'd done the usual college tour, we really were only comfortable with her being in Denver or Washington, D.C., where we had family that she knew and could turn to at holidays, or in times of feeling the separation of living on the opposite side of the globe from us and the world in which she grew up. My wife took her to get settled in at Denver University. I'm glad she wasn't around to see me especially that fall. That was the beginning of the roughest time. We were concerned about our daughter's adjustment and thankful Jane's sister Judy and her husband Ron were there for her. It was an arduous time for my wife and I compounded that considerably.

In my July visit with Dr. Lesser, we had discussed my continuing seizures and he had proposed that I taper off Lamictal and replace it with something new, an anti-seizure drug called Keppra. Keppra is a brand name for levetiracetam, and is described by its manufacturer and the FDA as an "adjunctive therapy for the treatment of Primary Generalized Tonic-Clonic seizures in patients with Idiopathic Generalized Epilepsy."[1] So this was an add-on to focus on major convulsive seizures and not those confined to one hemisphere. That sounded like a reasonable choice. His plan was I would begin by taking 250 milligrams of Keppra daily, then in weekly intervals increase the dose to 500 milligrams, 750, 1000 and up to 2000 and eventually 3000, which is the maximum recommended dosage in the FDA approval of the drug.[2] At the same time I could begin decreasing Lamictal by 100 milligrams weekly. He wrote in the report of our meeting, "If the Keppra does not control the patient's seizures or if he has side effects, we will next try Trileptal or Zonegran," and he also gave me a prescription for a year's worth of Keppra. That was how I was still getting much of my medicine, buying year's prescriptions and paying for them then submitting the receipts for payment to our

Singapore insurance company. He was dictating his notes into a Dictaphone, which he always did during our appointments, so a typist could make them part of a permanent record. As he was walking away, I heard him say "cc to Dr. Hui," in a reference to Dr. Lim Shih Hui. He had left quickly to get to another appointment or meeting but I rushed to catch him. I said that I'd heard him say "Dr. Hui," but that was incorrect. The doctor he was referring to was Chinese so his last name came first. His name was "Dr. Lim." Lesser looked a bit irritated and said that he knew that, which I imagine he did with his extensive travel and contacts, but it was an understandable mistake for those not familiar with Eastern cultures.

I didn't start the Keppra immediately, but waited until returning to Singapore. Jane had gone off with Anne to get her settled in college and the medicine transformation seemed to work out for a time when I began with the small dose of 250 milligrams and eliminated 100 milligrams of Lamictal. I continued and got all the way to 2000 milligrams of Keppra in later October. I don't remember whether I'd noticed anything much before then, but that seemed to be some sort of critical mass. I was hit by a barrage of side effects like never before.

Every epilepsy medication comes with a long list of possible gloomy side effects and perhaps with some I'd experienced limited reactions, particularly regarding alertness. This time it was like nearly everything on the list hit me at once. It was a debilitating experience. I had hallucinations, especially seeing the strange colored fabric of the drapes from my childhood days in my parents' home, framing whatever I was looking at. In some ways, I was becoming psychotic. Our home had a main floor and an upstairs, where we had our bedrooms. I not only stopped going to work, but for much of the time I refused to go down the stairs. I would stay in our bedroom and allow my anxieties to consume me in my own world. Our maid would bring me food and when Jane returned I could get down and look at the TV for a bit without paying much attention.

It was a desperate situation and I tried to contact Dr. Lesser, who returned my call when he was at work, which was the middle of the night in Singapore. I managed a brief conversation but was confused and failed to convey or understand anything. My wife and my sister became more involved so things happened. On October 24 Jane wrote to my sister, Patty, asking her to make connections with Johns Hopkins for directions. She copied my nephew Rick, a very knowledgeable young doctor, on the email. Her message began with a list of the current symptoms I had been exhibiting. These were anxiety, shakiness, confusion, clammy, feels hot and cold, feet and lower legs: very bad—can't feel, jumpy, not clear headed, twitchiness in face, feels like arches have collapsed or cramps in the bottom of the feet, hearing is weird, perceptions are questionable, voice is weak and he hears it inside his head, seizure today and last Friday (involved the right side of his face and voice), difficulty moving around, memory gaps, symptoms aren't improving.

I was clearly not much fun to be around and I wasn't sure I had control over who I was. Jane's message said that I was scared. She also said I didn't complain unless things were serious and that she'd always felt if I'd complained when I first got sick, I might not have any of the problems I have. I had gone to a doctor when I first got sick and she was away, but this comment might have been her recognition of what I'd become, how much of a burden on her it was that would only get worse.

My sister got in touch with Johns Hopkins and Dr. Lesser was out of the country. She spoke with a nurse named Sairyn, who worked for both Dr. Lesser and Dr. Krauss, the person who was covering Lesser's appointments until he returned in the second week of November. On Tuesday, October 25, the day after Jane wrote, Sairyn sent me an email with incredibly detailed instructions. He apparently had access to Dr. Lesser's records since he told me that Lesser had said if I had seizures or side effects from switching to Keppra, he wanted me to change to another drug, Trileptal. The transition plan he sent was 300 milligrams of Trileptal twice a day for three days then 600 twice a day. To accompany this I was to cut back on Keppra to 500 milligrams twice a day for three days, then none. He had attempted to send me a prescription for the Trileptal in Singapore but was unsuccessful so he sent it to my sister, who was collecting it at a pharmacy and sending it overnight to Singapore, which she did. He also said I should go to the emergency room if I continued to have seizures or side effects.

While I was still having side effects, I did not go to an emergency room. I was somewhat apprehensive about Sairyn's schedule which called for the elimination of my main medication in three days and wrote back expressing my concern. It is always recommended to avoid making abrupt changes with anti-seizure medications. It turned out the same was true with Keppra, according to the FDA.[3] There was more communication and my local doctor was involved. He recommended returning to Lamictal as my adjunct under the circumstances. There was also discussion of the need for a nerve test because of the decrease in feelings in my legs. A new schedule was worked out that wasn't quite as rushed.

I went off of Keppra over a one-week period, starting at 1000 milligrams per day and every other day taking 250 milligrams less. During the process, I was coherent enough to make my way to the hospital one day for a nerve test that confirmed again that I had neuropathy. On the last day in October, Sairyn sent me a message again to say that Dr. Krauss wanted me to get started on the Trileptal. By that time, I was within a day or so of being completely off Keppra and the strange things I'd been experiencing had nearly all faded away. In the first week of November, I returned to work and normalcy. My brief spell of insanity had ended, but the potency of the drugs we are prescribed was made very real to me. It was so great to have it over and get back to things familiar, getting up in the morning, going to work teaching classes, seeing people I knew.

At the end of school on that first week back on Friday I did what was my normal routine. Not long after the dismissal bell I made my way to the high school office which had an open area next to it to meet the students who had come to visit the leprosy home that week. Our small bus had to wait until all the school buses departed. It had been a bit of a stress coming back but I couldn't miss this. We made our uplifting visit, and while we visited the residents many of them gave me gifts of fruit. This was very common. Ever since they had come to expect me, some of them gave me gifts, which initially I attempted to refuse, but that was impolite. Often, the residents had been given quantities of fruit left over from fruit stands around the cities and were overwhelmed with it, so they passed much along as their way of welcoming. I began accepting all gifts, fruit and otherwise, and some other sponsors and several students also began to receive some. Upon returning to school we would bring what we had received into the high school office and leave it for Boni, the secretary, who would manage to distribute it to cleaners, guards, drivers and others when she returned to work on Monday.

This time, after getting in the office and leaving the food I started to have an aura. I didn't feel right. Not at all. I stepped into the open area next to the office, then I collapsed and began convulsing and it didn't stop. This was more than a grand mal seizure. It was November 7, only several days since I'd finished my episode with Keppra, and now I was in a state of status epilepticus.

So earlier that week my sanity seemed to have been at risk, but now it was my life. *Epilepsia* reported that status seizures were fatal in adults at a rate of 15–22 percent at this time,[4] though a study on a large group had found the number to be 32 percent.[5] That was an improvement due to pharmaceuticals and emergency care. That was to become an issue for me, since I would be making a life change and would spend months alone in an isolated mountain cabin where I could write. If I had a status seizure alone in isolated circumstances, I'd be on my own and the story would be different. The same *Epilepsia* article shed light on that, as it reported the mortality rate in 1880 before emergency services were as common or the appropriate drugs had been developed to stop seizures. The figure then was that 50 percent of the cases were fatal.[6] Brain damage was another concern with status seizures.

Someone called an ambulance and when it arrived, it backed right up the inclined stairs to the first floor before the first responders managed to load me in the back. Whether I had a brief lucid moment, or someone managed to reach Jane, I'm unsure. They did not head toward the nearest hospital, but one that was about the farthest away. It was Singapore General Hospital, a public hospital on the opposite side of Singapore where my doctor practiced.

I was in intensive care with no visitors allowed, other than my wife. My superintendent and his wife were informed and came to the hospital but were denied access to see me. In all, it was shaping up to be a tough week. I spent three days in the hospital where the care was outstanding. There was disagreement between the doctors on whether my stay should be extended, but my personal doctor, Dr. Lim, had final say and had me released.

I returned to work and began my experiment by adding Trileptal to the drug cocktail I was taking along with Topamax and Lamictal. While my neuropathy already provided some challenge to balance, the combination of drugs made matters worse. That was apparent a couple months later when the phone rang on the counter by our front entrance. I rushed from the couch to answer it with little awareness where my feet were and caught a toe on the corner of the frame of the couch. After the call, I looked at my toe. It turned at a right angle at the joint. It hurt and Jane and I considered what should be done. I remembered being with a friend and going to the emergency room after he dislocated a finger. When we arrived, they grabbed it and snapped it back in place and I thought perhaps I could do the same. We decided to go to the emergency room, where I saw an orthopedic surgeon. He not only yanked it straight but also inserted a wire straight up the toe to keep the joint from failing. I had to wear sandals to school for a time and my toe ended with a locked joint. That would interfere with one of my great pleasures, reflexology, but I would give them instructions to not try to bend or manipulate that toe.

Jane and I talked things over and it seemed like I might do better with less stress and more rest, as auras and minor seizures continued. I applied to become a part time teacher due to medical disability. Partial disability was something new at our school, but the provision was in our school's contract. Our Assistant Superintendent for Human Resources, Rhonda Norris, was very helpful in making arrangements with the insurance company and accumulating the many forms necessary for me to file about my medical history and with my doctors. Of all my doctors, only Dr. Lesser was asked to fill out extensive forms full of technical terms describing my health. I soon received approval and my teaching schedule for the next year would be three-fifths time. That meant I would continue to teach A.P. European History, a course on game theory, and another of Western Civilization or European History, depending on enrollment. Since our classes were "double block" or 90 minutes and met every other day, it also meant that every weekend would be three days. What I hoped for were the weeks when I went Tuesday–Friday because teachers' meetings were on Mondays and I could be at home for those, and Fridays were the leprosy home, so I always came to school at some point in any case.

That summer began with another visit to Dr. Lesser at Johns Hopkins. He again brought up the vagus nerve stimulator, and also drug prices. His advice was for me to buy them in Asia if they were brand name and less expensive, rather than in the United States to take them all back for the year. We also talked about adding Dilantin which had been successful very early on during my bout with epilepsy, but he didn't think it would be wise at that time. I was then on Trileptal, Topamax and Lamictal, and it was his hope to get me down to two medications, which would be a bit easier to balance and manage than three. That was apparently a long-term goal as his advice was that I taper off Lamictal 100 milligrams per week, while adding Zonegran at the same rate up to 400 milligrams per day. So my transition would still continue. That's another common experience for people with epilepsy, trying new drugs, always hoping the right one or combination will somehow be found. I took another fall in a cabin which required an ER visit in Steamboat Springs, Colorado. I was still having simple partial seizures and experimenting with new medicines.

I returned to teaching but things were becoming more difficult. When I moved around the campus, I usually kept one hand on a wall or a rail. In November, I returned to the United States and Johns Hopkins again. I'd been having weekly complex partial seizures and tried another new medicine, Zarontin, but with no benefit. We decided to give that up and return to Dilantin, going to 400 milligrams.

That got me by for a few months. In late April I met someone at a food court in a local market area. After having some fruit and coffee, I had an aura and it developed into a small seizure. That took him by surprise and he tried to be helpful. He walked me to a taxi stand and was waiting with me for a cab to arrive. That was when things really fell apart. I collapsed on the ground and began convulsing. Once again, it didn't stop. I was in status and an emergency case. He called an ambulance and then took my phone to find my wife's number and call her. The ambulance arrived and took me to National University Hospital.

When I regained consciousness, I was in intensive care. This was a different style of intensive care than others. Perhaps I'd been somewhere else originally, but from this time on I had the back-corner bed in a four-bed room. In the middle between me and the bed across from me was a desk where a nurse was permanently stationed to keep an eye on us. Visitors had chairs by our beds. This was apparently for serious cases and during my stay two of the others died and were replaced by new people. Jane was there regularly, often with her colleague Peggy, a good friend who had also come to the leprosy home regularly for a time. Peggy told me the doctors said the odds were against me surviving. Mine was going to be another available bed. This really looked like the "black blizzard" I feared.

I had a longer stay in the hospital this time than the previous status episode but felt in control when released. I soon met with Dr. Lim at Singapore General Hospital who would revise my medications again. He added Frisium, a benzodiazepine that I had tried for a bit in the 1990s in combination with different drugs. He left the Tegretol and Dilantin and completely eliminated any Lamictal or Zarontin. It was a three-drug combination that proved surprisingly helpful. One problem was that Frisium was not FDA approved, so not available in pharmacies in the United States. Since we didn't live in the United States that was not a major concern.

I returned and finished the year. It was clear it was time that I should find out whether not working would matter. In the fall, I applied for full disability as of the end of the year, effectively making that the last of my 37 years of teaching. I went to get the new forms, and the company said they weren't required. My previous forms had qualified me for full disability. Even though I hadn't taken it, my new status was official as of the end of the 2005-2006 school year. Coincidentally, Tom Schelling, my former teacher whose biography I'd been writing and whose ideas provided the basis for a course I taught, was awarded the Nobel Prize in Economics in 2005 during that final teaching year. That brought new interest to the book I'd been working on and gave me a focus for using my time when I'd leave my lifelong work in the spring.

21

Difficulties Leaving

So that's what I was, disabled. What does the dictionary say that is? It means "impaired or limited by a physical, mental, cognitive, or developmental condition."[1] And Lesser had said I was handicapped, which the dictionary similarly described as "having a physical or mental disability" along with saying the word is "sometimes offensive."[2] I was just an impaired, unemployed person, while the people I'd known for years continued to work. I kept busy with writing and attending some events as well as always showing up at the school on Fridays to go to the leprosy home, and on occasion see old friends. It wasn't the same when I wasn't part of it anymore but that was all right. There were soon new things.

Even though I was not working, we remained in Singapore for eight more years and I had a couple of books released. My wife continued to teach and our daughter returned and became a teacher at the same school, Singapore American School. My seizures were under better control since the final combination of medications worked out by Dr. Lim, though I still had partial seizures from time to time. On occasion, these would cause me to fall. I had a general practice doctor, the very special Dr. Georgia Lee, who suggested that I should start using a walking stick. It was not so much because I needed it, but she said because of the way I walked with my neuropathy and all the medication, people seeing me were likely to think I was drunk. I hadn't thought of that, but it was obvious she was right as usual. I got a metal one in a hospital shop and following that it became a hobby, collecting different walking sticks from around the world. It soon became difficult to navigate without one.

Dr. Lee also asked if I would be willing to try local medicine for my neuropathy since nothing else was working. I was, and she arranged an appointment at Tan Tok Seng Hospital with a practitioner of Chinese medicine who gave me an exam, but said he had nothing to offer. That and my osteoporosis were becoming problems. Those who take anti-seizure medication for long periods of time are likely to develop osteoporosis, since the medicines leach calcium from the bones.[3] It turned up on a scan I had for something else and I began taking medicine for it, but the condition would not go away. That problem revealed itself for me soon.

While Jane continued to work, I spent longer periods in the mountains of Colorado at the cabin owned by my sister and her husband. I'd go in May before school ended and remain until September after it had begun again. It was extremely secluded and a great place for writing while enjoying the surroundings. It was a somewhat risky place. While I had quite good control, I really didn't have total control over the abnormal electric activity in my head that could cause seizures. I would be alone for up to weeks without visitors, and only saw people when I walked to one of the two cabins within a mile to visit the people who remained on "the hill" as we called it for the entire summer and into the fall. I knew that in these conditions, if I had a serious seizure while in the cabin or on a hike, especially a status seizure or multiple seizures which had happened five times previously, and had needed emergency medical treatment, I might just be found dead eventually when someone arrived. Those "black blizzards" were still lurking in there and whether they would cross the threshold from remaining on one side, in one area, to become a full-blown storm again would only be known if it happened. I had decided that it couldn't dictate how I lived my life.

In 2011 I was alone at the cabin and watching the NBA (National Basketball Association) championships, hoping Miami would lose. I had a pot pie in the microwave and had just opened a beer when the phone rang. It was one of my neighbors, Faith, and while we were talking the timer went off for the microwave. What happened next is unclear and I do not recall that I had any type of seizure, but perhaps my neuropathy played a role in the fall I took. I dropped the phone. Fortunately Faith knew of my epilepsy and called a young man who trimmed trees at our cabin and worked for her and asked him to drive his truck up and check on me. What I first noticed when I hit the ground was that my forearm appeared swollen, which seemed too soon. Shortly after, a truck was there and I was driven to the emergency room in Estes Park, a small mountain town near the cabin. After doing an X-ray the ER doctor talked to me and contacted their orthopedic specialist. My arm wasn't swollen, it had become more than an inch shorter than the other because everything had been "shattered" and both bones of my forearm, the radius and ulna, had completely broken and the bones were overlapping, sitting on top of each other. There were also many other small breaks. I was hospitalized briefly then taken to an operating room when the orthopedic surgeon arrived. He did what was as unpleasant a procedure as I've experienced, called "repositioning." Though I was given some medication it had no effect. Perhaps they were being cautious because of my many medications. I was placed on a table and held by four nurses while the doctor grabbed my broken arm and sharply yanked it to pull the bones back into position. He then repeated the procedure as I was held. Then I was brought to a room and my wife, who had just arrived from Singapore, showed up at the hospital with her sister. The next morning, I had four hours of surgery that involved putting in two metal plates and 19 bolts plus some cadaver bone. That brought the total amount of metal in me to five plates, 37 bolts, all titanium, so nothing set off the detectors at airports. The operation was followed by physical therapy and I regained remarkable use of my left hand.

Our daughter had returned to Singapore and worked in school, earned a teacher's certificate and become an elementary teacher where she attended school and her parents taught. She met another teacher and they were married. In time, they had a daughter, our first grandchild, Mya. While I was allowed to see Mya on most Sundays, first at our apartment or theirs, then at the American Club, I was only allowed to hold her briefly and often given instructions about how it should be done. There always seemed to be a degree of worry about what might happen if I were responsible for Mya with my precarious health and the fragile young girl. Two years later she had a second child, Tai, and that remained the situation. I was still having problems, but they were minor. Time passed and I had no seizures involving convulsions or loss of consciousness.

My sister and her husband came to visit Singapore, which they had done previously. While they were there, we took a cruise on the Singapore River, during which I had a complex partial seizure and fell, making a mess. It was preceded by an aura. I suppose my daughter's fears were justified. Having a fall when I had a partial seizure was unusual, but a problem. My usual response when I felt one was to find a place to sit or lean against a wall, since they were usually brief, then wait for them to pass.

During one of my summer stays at the cabin I had my prescription refilled shortly before to have plenty of medication to last until my return to Singapore. My habit by that time was to have our maid fill the daily packets of medication and put them in baggies that contained 30 or about a month's worth in each so I could take a few plus an extra in case there was some problem along the way. I still had some that I'd been using from a previous prescription when I left, then I got to Colorado and began using the recently prescribed pills. Initially I paid little attention but then noticed that what was supposed to be Frisium looked

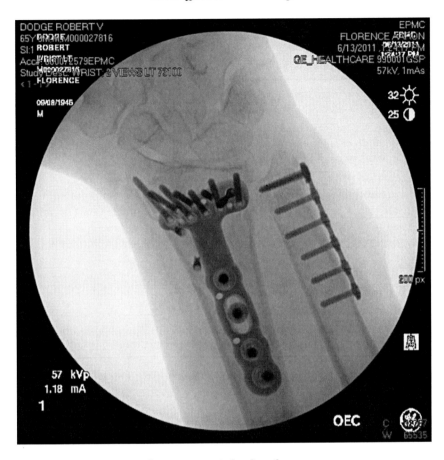

Implants to repair broken forearm.

different. Upon closer inspection, I saw that it was not Clobazam, which is Frisium, but Clonazepam. Very similar names and both were benzodiazepines, and prescribed for epilepsy. Both come as small white pills but there was a different letter on them. I sent an email to Dr. Lim in Singapore and he asked me to come in immediately after returning. When I did, he was extremely apologetic and said someone else wanted to see me. Outside was the hospital's director of its pharmacies who also apologized profusely and took me down to the main pharmacy by the clinics, where there were always about 100 or more people waiting to be served. I was immediately given a new prescription and I said thanks. I suspect they feared I was going to make an issue of this and possibly write to the newspaper or complain publicly in some other way.

It had worked out fine, but pointed out a real problem. A study done over the course of a year in a hospital where there were 7,400 prescriptions dispensed to patients found a 2.5 percent error rate in filling the prescriptions.[4] Fortunately, there was a second layer of screening and these errors were either caught by dispensing pharmacists or by nurses before they were administered.[5] They noted that poor handwriting was a "major source of error" in why incorrect prescriptions were dispensed.[6] While that could certainly remain a problem at numerous smaller practices and clinics, there are many larger facilities where things are done by computer and this should rarely be an issue anymore. Still, as I had learned, it is wise for the patient to look carefully at his prescription both before and after it is filled.

At another appointment with Dr. Lim following that he performed a simple test. I just sat and stared forward as he stood in front of me and lowered a finger from above my head near my face and asked when I could see it. He did this in several different locations, but when he lowered from above the left side of my left eye I failed to respond until his finger was directly in front of my eye. He ordered a test by an ophthalmologist. That test was done eye by eye individually. In turn, in a dark room and under a loose hood, each eye held open by a device while the other was closed. I looked at a dark screen directly in front of my face. I held a grip that had a button on the top, and every time I saw a flash of light appear briefly, I pushed the button. These were like brief views of one star in a very dark sky that appeared randomly anywhere in a 360° area. It wasn't a long test but there was a computer printout of the results. In the entire upper left quadrant of my vision I had absolutely no vision. I was one-quarter blind. This was the "pie in the sky" I'd been repeatedly warned of during my brain surgeries. Since I'm always aware of what I look at which is straight ahead, I had never realized what I wasn't seeing. Any thoughts I'd had of ever driving again were extinguished after seeing that test result. To me, my vision remained completely normal, but how easily I could miss seeing something and become a hazard to others.

Eventually, it was getting near time to return to the United States. Our school adopted a mandatory retirement policy, so my wife would be required to stop working in Singapore. There had been one major problem, which was my medicine. Things were satisfactory with the prescription I was on, the three-drug mixture of Frisium, Topamax, Dilantin. Frisium, which was a brand name for clobazam, hadn't been available in America because the FDA had not approved it. Dr. Lesser told me he could get it through his connections at the United Nations, where the pharmacy had to have drugs available from countries all around the world. That seemed like a tenuous connection to depend on.

Things came together at the right time. Frisium was approved by the FDA and released in the United States under the name Onfi. In 2014, we left Singapore after 31 years to return to the United States and chose Denver, Jane's twin sister's home. Our daughter's family moved to Doha in Qatar. Initially my wife spent a considerable amount of time in Doha helping out with the grandchildren so Anne and her husband could begin their new jobs. They eventually got a maid but the process took more time than they expected. As their first school year was coming to

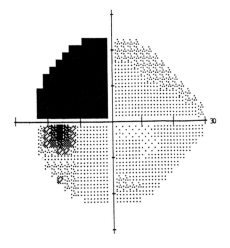

Computer image of vision in left eye.

an end, Anne's incredibly fit husband died tragically while working out in the compound gym. Since no foul play was involved there was no autopsy. My brother-in-law arranged for a former student of his to perform one upon the body's arrival in the United States and it was found the cause of death was an exceptionally large brain aneurysm that would only be discovered when it burst. Our daughter, Anne, was now a young widow with two small children. I kept writing and had other books released. I also made visits to Anne's family on their compound in Doha and we used the opportunity of traveling there to spend time in London and Paris.

Once we were back in the United States, we needed health care and enrolled in Medicare. I got all my prescriptions after paying $3,400 annually, then the remainder was paid by the government. But I also made a discovery about pharmaceutical companies in the United States that was very disturbing. While I only had to pay some of my costs and the government picked up most of the bill, still, it was hard to understand. There have since been more shocking stories that have made the news and attracted attention to pharmaceutical companies in exploiting people's need for prescriptions to make profits. Their ability to charge whatever prices they wanted since their customers would have to pay, or they had insurance, really brought out the greed in these companies.

How I discovered it was I'd reached a certain stability by taking Frisium (clobazam) which I got in 10 milligram pills and took four per day. A receipt I retained from Singapore in 2010 was for 120 tablets of Frisium at a regular public pharmacy chain for $38.76 Singapore dollars. Converting that at the exchange rate of the time and reducing the number to 100 tablets, the cost would have been $23.75 in U.S. dollars, and price per tablet in Singapore was $.34 Singapore currency which was 25 U.S. cents. Then we came to America. The price for 100 tablets of 10 milligram tablets listed online $2,309.28,[7] and the price per tablet is above $23.00. The same company, Lundbeck, was the manufacturer of both products. The same pills, same strength, from the same company were 95 times more expensive in the U.S than in Singapore. I got them for $2,626.89 per month for four 10 milligram daily pills through our Kaiser health plan so the identical medication that was $.25 per tablet in Singapore cost $21.89 each from the Kaiser Pharmacy. It could have been somewhat more reasonable through a Canadian pharmacy using a generic drug but it just made me wonder how there could be such a difference. The United States wasn't 95 times as expensive as Singapore so they hadn't lowered prices there to compensate for the poverty. It is really the opposite, as Singapore ranked with Hong Kong and Paris as tied for the most expensive city in the world by BBC News in March of 2019.[8]

At one point, I expressed my concerns over the high prices of anti-epileptic drugs to Dr. Lesser and asked his opinion on using generic substitutes to lower the costs. He had instructed me at the time to buy brand name medicine and sent a study that compared emergency hospital visits due to epilepsy. It showed that the highest rate was by people using mixed generics, followed by those who used one generic and stayed with it, and the least by those with brand name drugs. Another analysis at the time of my first operations concluded, "This study supports the argument against generic prescribing for epilepsy. It suggests that the small amount of money saved by generic prescribing is outweighed by negative health gain for the person with epilepsy."[9] Lesser said at the time that while the active ingredients were the same, there were differences in the chalks or other mixing substance, or the capsule used as a container that could impact the rate of absorption of the medicine.

When we settled in Denver our health care group was Kaiser and I learned that like most large groups, their pharmacy automatically supplied generics. I was going to see if I could request originals, but when I sent a message to Dr. Lesser, he replied that the generic for Onfi was fine to use. He was like that. For many years following my surgery and after I stopped having appointments with him, I still sent him emails to ask questions about my care and what I should do. There was always an auto-reply but in nearly every case he would write a response within one day. I sometimes thought perhaps he felt a little guilty that he'd given me advice and planned my four brain surgeries that had imposed considerable discomfort and cost. But I was still having seizures that in some ways seemed like they'd gotten worse, with the status seizures. I realize mine was not the typical experience and that the evidence is clear that surgery for epilepsy has commonly been a beneficial procedure.[10] That may have had nothing to do with it, but 20 years after having had surgery, then seeing him for expensive followup appointments, he was providing me with immediate advice and answers without charge, and his expertise was recognized by all, so I really appreciated it.

While I have no doubt that Dr. Lesser was correct in his comment on Onfi now having satisfactory generic versions, perhaps I should have asked him a different question. I did know when the generic became available, but only that we returned to the United States shortly after it had received FDA approval. When I first ordered it in my memory the price was very high. Every time I ordered a refill it was listed on the pharmacy website as "Onfi (clobazam)." I believed I was ordering the brand name product originally and realized that the price was later reduced. My number of simple partial seizures has increased since 2018, causing some falls. Up to that time I'd done considerable overseas travel both with my wife and on my own. I thought I was getting brand name until a conversation with a pharmacist while picking up a prescription. He said that everything they dispensed was a generic version of the medication. They had begun dispensing generic clobazam in 2018 and nobody had informed me. According to *Epilepsy & Behavior* in Colorado it is required to get a patient's permission before switching epilepsy medication from brand name to generic.[11] If you aren't told, you don't know.

Of course, it was an economic decision by Kaiser to rely entirely on generic drugs and it could be argued that it benefited patients by reducing costs. A 2016 review of the many academic studies of the effectiveness of brand name versus generic drugs for epilepsy patients recommend that "well-controlled epileptic patients should avoid switching from brand-to-generic products"[12] as well as making any other switches. It was never disclosed to me as a patient that when my prescription said Onfi it meant generic Onfi. Whether pharmacies even inform doctors of such changes and when they occur is a question, as is whether patients who are adjusted to being on a medication should be informed of the change from brand name to generic or from one generic to another, since the evidence is there are risks to their health that they should be aware of.

It turns out that the use of generics to save money on epilepsy medications by large providers so they can save money can lead to real problems. A good example is one medicine I've used more than any other, Dilantin, which is phenytoin. I was on it when we first moved to England

and received it through the National Health Services, or NHS. In Britain, where there is national healthcare, there is a charge of 9£ per prescription, which is currently just under $12, regardless of what medicine is prescribed. This may be refunded or exempted in some cases, while medicines are free in Scotland and Wales. What is called Dilantin, even though generics are being dispensed, is very widely used, so the NHS had long bought large supplies from pharmaceutical companies, then their opportunism and greed set in. Pfizer, the massive drug company, was the main supplier of the generic version of Dilantin for the NHS. They were fined $106 million by the government for overcharging the NHS. Flynn Pharma, a distributor that supplied a smaller amount, was fined $6.5 million for making a 2600 percent increase in the product used by 48,000 patients in the U.K between 2012 and 2013.[13] During that year NHS spending on Dilantin generics rose from £2 million to £50 million.[14] Big pharma got caught that time.

22

Issues Back in the U.S.A.

In the spring of 2014 we had permanently settled in the United States after our 35 years as expatriates. It wasn't for a visit but as a residence and I wasn't sure whether I had a long retirement to look forward to. Having epilepsy on average led to a reduced life expectancy of two years if it was cryptogenic or idiopathic, meaning it had no obvious cause, or up to 10 years if it was symptomatic, meaning it came from an injury to the brain.[1] I fell into both categories, having been described in medical reports as having idiopathic epilepsy, since it has not been fully responsive to medication and the cause is speculative, and also having medical reports frequently state that it resulted from having encephalitis, which injured my brain as defined as symptomatic. It appears that symptomatic has been used to refer more to injuries than illnesses and especially references seizures from brain tumors, strokes or serious head injuries. In any case, it didn't matter and whatever would happen, there would be no reason to act any differently.

Transportation is a very common problem for people with epilepsy and though I did not intend to drive in Denver, there were wide open spaces and open roads with very few vehicles when we headed from Denver to the mountains. It seemed like it might be safe to resume driving in those situations, where I really only needed to look straight ahead and stay on the road. Living in Denver was going to be a challenge. The metropolitan area was spread out over a large area and public transportation wasn't readily available, like in Singapore or London. I learned that laws had changed considerably since the time I was first diagnosed and automatically had my license removed and it required a year without a seizure, certified by my doctor, then I had to apply for a new license and go through the process of taking the test to get one. The situation had become less strict, though it varied from state to state. That had changed, so that only six states required doctors to report patients who were diagnosed with epilepsy,[2] but all epilepsy patients were expected to self-report their condition to their local department of motor vehicles. Suspension of driving time following a seizure had been reduced to three or six months, with some exceptions. North Dakota no longer had doctor reporting and its six-month license suspension could be appealed for evaluation to be reduced to three months. Colorado, our new home, also had no requirement of doctor reporting but had no specified period of license suspension. Its only requirement was a medical update at the discretion of the motor vehicles department.[3] A 2010 study found that two-thirds of people with epilepsy thought they could safely drive, while only one-third had been counseled on the risks of driving.[4] Of those counseled, they found a significant minority continued to drive after being advised not to, and some were involved in seizure-related accidents.[5] Not driving was going to be more of an inconvenience than it had been, and my new doctor offered to have me take a vision test to see whether I would be eligible for a provisional license. Much as not driving was a loss of freedom, I had adjusted to that and didn't want to take any chance especially of doing harm to others. Uber had come to Denver, soon followed by Lyft, so things became generally manageable.

Not long after arriving I was in a local bookstore and saw a *National Lampoon* collection that I thought might be entertaining. It included a cartoon of a mechanical pony for children with a slot for a coin and a sign saying, "PONY RIDE 25 Cents." On the ground, next to the pony was a man on his hands and knees with a sign propped up in front of him that read, "RIDE AN EPILEPTIC 35 Cents."[6] Welcome back.

While this was an old cartoon the attitudes about people with epilepsy were not greatly improved. The Americans with Disabilities Act, the ADA that had passed in 1991, was a major step forward that included those with epilepsy among its many beneficiaries who were granted some rights and recognition. It represented that some were aware that people in their communities needed a legal space carved out, a space that said we are not "others," but while some things may be more difficult for us, we are members of society and deserve to be included. How welcoming people were to those of us with epilepsy was a different story. The U.S. Centers for Disease Control did a survey in 2013 about attitudes toward people with epilepsy to compare it with one they had done previously. They selected over 11,000 people for initial interviews and out of those did a further survey to get data matched to the general population by sex, age, household income, race/ethnicity and household size.[7] Their research showed that people had increased in confidence that people with epilepsy could work 40-hour-per-week jobs successfully. But "on the other hand, our study also suggests that many adults continue to express concern about being around or interacting with people with epilepsy. More troubling, this level of fear and avoidance was significantly higher in 2013 than in 2005. Adults in 2013 were significantly less likely to disagree with not wanting to date, with not wanting to let their child date, or with not wanting to work with people with epilepsy, as well as feeling uncomfortable around or being afraid to be alone with people with epilepsy."[8]

One thing epilepsy organizations did to combat this was to proclaim the achievements of people with epilepsy and how they had impacted the course of history. A recurring theme highlighted by the recognition of the greatness of Julius Caesar has been that having epilepsy is associated with genius and there is inspiration, divine or otherwise, during seizures, that inspires artists or allows for insightful breakthroughs in creative thoughts that impact society. One study noted that this connection dates back to ancient times and that Socrates suggested poets must rely on madness for creative expression, while Aristotle maintained that great genius only existed with some madness and that all extraordinary men tend to be melancholic.[9] This study found that the common factor among creative achievers was that they were the products of distress, whether broken homes, alcoholism, sexual problems, or physical handicaps including specifically epilepsy. These were all conditions that led to isolation. The sense of isolation that these people who were "others" felt promoted a tendency to work alone and develop a unique knowledge and skill which was the essence of creativity.[10]

This idea appears to have gained credence during the Romantic Era of the early 1800s, as genius had been considered a form of insanity from ancient times up to then, according to a *History of Ideas* publication on epilepsy and genius.[11] This paper discussed Dostoevsky's epilepsy and his use of it in three major novels, *The Idiot*, *The Devils*, and *The Brothers Karamazov*, and how it was used in the late 1800s to relate the saintly and criminal qualities it manifests. Epilepsy was associated with criminal behavior at the time, and Dostoevsky told a friend that after a seizure, "I feel like a great criminal."[12] The author remarked that epilepsy has been associated with both crime and religion, noting both Mohammed and Jesus have been alleged to have been epileptics.[13]

The Romantic connection ended with the eugenics movement and people with epilepsy were reduced to being considered mentally defective, as had been the case previously with the many who were not the exceptionally talented. Even so, the relationship of epilepsy and genius occurred during the height of the Eugenics movement in the place where it started. A comment entitled "Illness and Intellect" appeared in a 1912 issue of *The British Medical Journal*. The author wrote in response to an article on how few people with epilepsy succeed had cited evidence from the War Office. Its reply was "How on earth did Hannibal and Marlborough and Wellington manage? Probably, if you examined the evidence, you would find it positive that they had epilepsy as that Caesar and Mahomet had. I see now why Luther was such an effective force in his prime."[14]

Also during time the of Eugenics movement Mathew Woods, a doctor who had spent 25 years working with patients who had epilepsy and was not only a member of the American Medical Association, but also the Philadelphia Psychiatric Association for the Study of Epilepsy and Epileptics, wrote a book called *In Spite of Epilepsy*. Its subtitle was *Being a Review of the Lives of Three Great Epileptics,—Julius Caesar, Mohammed, Lord Byron,—The Founders Respectively of an Empire, a Religion, and a School of Poetry*.[15]

In more recent times there have been considerable claims about epilepsy and influential people from history and the present. A list from *Disabled World's* website of prominent figures who had epilepsy includes, among others, Alexander the Great, Pythagoras, Socrates, Aristotle, Julius Caesar, Hannibal, Alfred the Great, Michelangelo, Leonardo Da Vinci, Martin Luther, Sir Isaac Newton, Peter the Great, Handel, Napoleon, Lord Byron, James Madison, Edgar Allan Poe, Tchaikovsky, Alfred Nobel, Vincent van Gogh, Theodore Roosevelt, and, more recently, Danny Glover and Prince.[16] The world's only epilepsy museum, located in Kork, Germany, also includes in its gallery of famous people with epilepsy Hercules, King Saul, St. Paul, Joan of Arc, Lenin, Pope Pius IX.[17]

While these are encouraging to those of us with epilepsy and no doubt that is the reason for posting such claims, academic journals find they rest on little support in documents. John Hughes did a study that was reported in *Epilepsy & Behavior* in 2005 that examined the supporting claims about famous people having had epilepsy.[18] He described the evidence and symptoms of many, among them Dante, Aristotle, Hannibal, Alfred the Great, Joan of Arc, Leonardo da Vinci, Michelangelo, Cardinal Richelieu, Pascal, Louis XIII of France, Moliére, Sir Isaac Newton, William of Orange, Jonathan Swift, Handel, William Pitt, Samuel Johnson, Rousseau, Madison, Beethoven, Lord Byron, Tolstoy, Lewis Carroll, Alfred Nobel, Tchaikovsky, Agatha Christie, Truman Capote, Richard Burton and found no convincing evidence any had epilepsy. Some had seizures, but they were more likely from other causes such as alcohol withdrawal, poison or a number of specified conditions.[19]

Contrary to this, the *Journal of Medical Biography* examined far fewer people but concluded "there is considerable evidence to suggest that Socrates, St Paul and Joan of Arc all experienced epileptic attacks during their lives."[20]

Perhaps some of the most influential people of all time or currently living are victims of epilepsy. The Epilepsy Foundation reports that currently there are 64 million people in the world with epilepsy, including 3.4 million in the United States,[21] so it will not be surprising if some accomplish great things. It may well be that epilepsy has not provided insights to change the course of history and it is not necessary to advance that claim to defend oneself from assumptions of being mentally or artistically inferior. People with epilepsy come in all categories. "Purple Rain" singer and seven-time Grammy winner Prince acknowledged in a 2009 interview that he had suffered from epilepsy throughout his life.[22] Supreme Court Chief Justice John Roberts fell after having his second seizure on July 30, 2007,[23] the standard definition of epilepsy.

What is clear is that people are uncomfortable around us. That was another reason some people tried to remain in denial. Perhaps that is why the claims of people from the past are not well documented and remain controversial. I realize it remains true in my case. Jane told me I made her family nervous. That's understandable. Was it the epilepsy or what the treatment does to me? Perhaps it didn't matter. I know it wasn't that much fun to be around me, especially when I was aware of a degree of tension from people feeling worried that I might have a seizure in their presence and they would be responsible for what happened next. It was a concern which was legitimate, but it reduced me somewhat to withdraw or become defensive for being what I was.

Things were not really improving and falling became more of an issue, which also made people nervous. There was one at the end of a walk I often took to get exercise. I'd reached the door of our apartment building but felt things going wrong. I had a partial seizure and collapsed. Friendly neighbors helped me up and to our apartment. When I told Jane that my foot continued to hurt, she thought we should go to an emergency room. It turned out I'd broken my ankle. So I was in a cast and using a walker for a time then going through physical therapy. I had falls in a number of places, sometimes following very brief seizures, from tripping due to my neuropathy, at other times because of my lack of balance that was at least partially from the large doses of medication.

One happened at home when we were to go to an event and I fell in the bathroom. My lower back hurt, but I continued to get prepared. Again, it was Jane who insisted that if I was in pain then it was serious, so she drove me to an emergency room. This time I'd broken six ribs, one of which had punctured a lung that deflated.

So I found myself not very sociable as life still presented some difficulties and also because I had turned inward. It suited my situation since I'd become a writer so enjoyed time alone and often ignored others around me. There were local organizations I discovered that were interesting and that I had begun participating in but much of my life was quite solitary. My wife had her own life and friends which was very active and fulfilling and we still shared time together for our regular home life.

People with epilepsy are often depressed. Some psychiatrists and neurologists put the correlation between the two conditions at 55 percent.[24] In his paper "Depression in Epilepsy" Dr. Marco Mula wrote that mood disorders were most frequently encountered that paired epilepsy and depression, were associated with poor quality of life, severe seizures, side effects of epilepsy medications and poor outcomes after epilepsy surgery.[25] I might seem to meet some of his criteria. He added that depression and temporal lobe epilepsy share a disruption in the same brain networks,[26] and that suicide represents 11.5 percent of all causes of death in epilepsy.[27] I didn't think of myself as depressed, but realize there have been deflating and depressing aspects of this life with the "black blizzards" in my head that I always know are there, regardless of what the situation is. Every day I'm reminded by the many pills and the schedule of when to take them that my life is in the control of this condition. Even though the operations seem to have taken away the original trigger, being set off by music, to the present I become nervous when music is very loud or jarring and my panic reactions immediately begin. There are enough partial seizures which my medication combination manages to control, but at times I can feel they have spread a bit farther than others. I've always had the idea that at some point the condition was going to win. That's not fatalism, just years of trying so many things and still not being free.

Rather than depressed I am often very happy. I keep that largely to myself as well. I'm still getting by fine, while many people have so much more to deal with. My problems are manageable and mainly frustrations. In 2018 the opportunity presented itself to make a brief visit to Singapore and once again visit those whose lives kept my difficulties in perspective, the victims of leprosy.

My major negative feeling is one that I share with many others

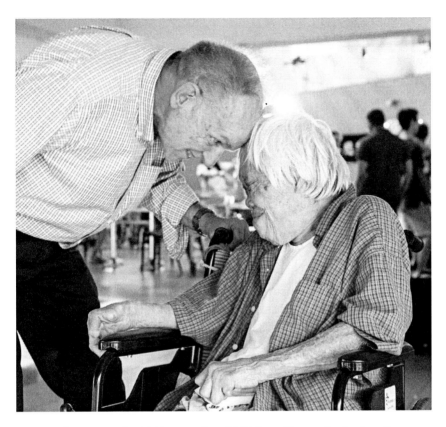

Visit to Singapore in 2018, greeting SILRA resident who had epilepsy as well as leprosy.

in my condition. That is how much of the time I feel that I am a burden.[28] This is especially true in my relationship with my wife but it is a continually recurring theme in interactions with family, friends, strangers. With my wife, I realize how much of her life has been spent on looking after me in some way, whether it was in emergency situations or just day to day life. There is the problem, especially now that we are back in the United States, of getting groceries, plus other details of daily living that have become her responsibility. I am less involved than she and often more of an obligation than help when it comes to taking care of the grandchildren and keeping up while going crowded places.

The goal for people with epilepsy is that they will achieve control on monotherapy, and some do. I've been through four brain surgeries and been on Phenobarbital, Dilantin, Mysoline, Tegretol, Depakote, Depakene, Epilim, Frisium, Lamictal, Neurontin, Topamax, Keppra, Trileptal,

Zonegran, and Zarontin as well as Onfi for seizure control along with Ativan and Diazapam for controlling situations that could become emergencies. So after 15 different drugs there has been no magic bullet and I remain on a fairly successful combination of three while still using Ativan on occasion.

The "black blizzard" remains in my head and on my mind. All of that for not swatting one mosquito long ago.

Chapter Notes

Chapter 2

1. Pat Phillips, "Tripartite Global Initiative on Epilepsy Announced," *Journal of the American Medical Association*, Vol. 278, Iss. 11, September 17, 1997, 885. Also, E.M. Airaksinen. R. Matilainen, T. Mononen, K. Mustonsen, J. Partanen, V. Jokela and P. Halonen, "A Population-Based Study on Epilepsy in Mentally-Retarded Children," *Epilepsia*, Vol. 41, No. 9, September 2000, 1214–1220.

2. Robert S. Fisher and Ilo Leppik, "Debate: When Does a Seizure Imply Epilepsy?" *Epilepsia*, December 5, 2008, 7.

3. "What Is Epilepsy?" *Epilepsy Foundation*, https://www.epilepsy.com/learn/about-epilepsy-basics/what-epilepsy.

4. Roger S. Fisher, Walter van Emde Boas, Warren Blume, Christiåan Elger, Pierre Genton, Phillip Lee, and Jerome Engel, Jr., "Epileptic Seizures and Epilepsy: Definitions Proposed by the International League Against Epilepsy (ILAE) and the International Bureau for Epilepsy (IBE)," *Epilepsia*, Vol. 6, No. 4, April 2005, 477.

5. Robert S. Fisher, Carlos Acevedo, Alexis Arzimanoglou, Alicia Bogacz, J. Helen Cross, Christian E. Elger, Jerome Engel Jr, Lars Forsgren, Jacqueline A. French, Mike Glynn, Dale C. Hesdorffer, B.I. Lee, Gary W. Mathern, Solomon L. Moshe, Emilio Perucca, Ingrid E. Scheffer, Torbjörn Tomson, Masako Watanabe, and Samuel Wiebe, "ILEA Special Report: A Practical Clinical Definition of Epilepsy," *Epilepsia*, Vol. 55, No. 4, April 14, 2014, 477.

6. Lois G. Kim, Tony L. Johnson, Anthony G. Marson, David W. Chadwick,

"Prediction of Risk of Seizure Recurrence After a Single Seizure and Early Epilepsy: Further Results from the MESS Trial," *Lancet*, Vol. 5, Iss. 4, April 2006.

7. Fisher et al., "ILEA Special Report," 477.

8. Fisher and Leppik, "Debate," 8.

9. Roger S. Fisher et al., "Epileptic Seizures and Epilepsy," 472.

10. "The Epilepsies and Seizures: Hope Through Research," *NIH*, https://www.ninds.nih.gov/Disorders/Patient-Caregiver-Education/Hope-Through-Research/Epilepsies-and-Seizures-Hope-Through, December 30, 2019.

11. William C. Shiel Jr., "Medical Definition of Epilepsy," *MedicineNet*, https://www.medicinenet.com/script/main/art.asp?articlekey=3285, December 4, 2018.

12. "What Is Epilepsy?" *Epilepsy Foundation*.

13. "Epilepsy," *World Health Organization*, https://www.who.int/news-room/fact-sheets/detail/epilepsy, June 20, 2019.

14. Jerome Engel, Jr., Timothy A. Pedley, *Epilepsy: A Comprehensive Textbook* (Philadelphia: Lippincott Williams & Wilkins, 2008), 1.

15. "Epilepsy," *Mayo Clinic*, https://www.mayoclinic.org/diseases-conditions/ epilepsy/symptoms-causes/syc-20350093.

16. Fisher et al., "ILEA Special Report," 476.

17. Romel W. Mackelprang and Richard O. Salsgiver, "People with Disabilities and Social Work: Historical and Contemporary Issues," *Social Work*, Vol. 41, No. 1, January 1996, 10.

18. Irene M. Elliot, Lucyna Lach, Mary Lou Smith, " I Just Want to Be Normal: A

Qualitative Study Exploring How Children and Adolescents View the Impact of Intractable Epilepsy on Their Quality of Life," *Epilepsy & Behavior*, Vol. 7, Iss. 4, December1, 2005, 669–670.

19. Judith Welch Wegner, "Antodiscrimination Model Reconsidered: Ensuring Equal Opportunity Without Respect to Handicap Under Section 504 of the Rehabilitation Act of 1973," *Cornell Law Review*, Vol. 69, No. 401, 403, N 2, 1984.

20. Arlene Mayerson, "The History of the ADA: A Movement Perspective," *Disability Rights and Education Fund*, https://www.ohio.k12.ky.us/userfiles/1173/Classes/8431/The%20History%20of%20the%20ADA.pdf, 1992.

21. "Our Documents—Civil Rights Act 1964," 1https://www.ourdocuments.gov/doc.php?flash=true&doc=97.

22. As quoted in Wegner, "Antodiscrimination Model Reconsidered," 403.

23. Melissa Fanulari, " The Effects of a Disability on Labor Market Performance: The Case of Epilepsy," *Southern Economic Journal*, Vol. 58, No. 4, April 1992, 1072.

24. Tom DeLeire, "The Wage and Employment Effects of the Americans with Disabilities Act," *Journal of Human Resources*, Vol. 35, No. 4, Autumn 2000, 699.

25. Fanulari, "The Effects of a Disability," 1080.

26. *Ibid.*, 1081.

27. *Ibid.*, 1084.

28. George H.W. Bush, "Remarks of President George Bush at the Signing of the Americans with Disabilities Act," https://www.eeoc.gov/eeoc/history/35th/videos/ada_signing_text.html, July 26, 1990.

29. "Americans with Disabilities Act," https://legcounsel.house.gov/Comps/Americans%20With%20Disabilities%20Act%20Of%201990.pdf.

Chapter 3

1. Fred H. Gage and Alysson R. Muotri, "What Makes Each Brain Unique," *Scientific American*, March 2012, 25.

2. "The Brain Is the 'Most Complex Thing in the Universe,'" *BBC* online, May 29, 2012.

3. See Hartmut Wekerle, "Immune Protection of the Brain," *Journal of Infectious Diseases*, Vol. 186, Supp. 2, December 1, 2002.

4. Description of brain anatomy from "Anatomy of the Brain," *American Association of Neurosurgical Surgeons*, https://www.aans.org/en/Patients/Neurosurgical-Conditions-and-Treatments/Anatomy-of-the-Brain; Matthew Hoffman, "Human Anatomy," *WebMD*, http://www.webmd.com/brain/picture-of-the-brain#1; Catherine Zuckerman, "The Human Brain Explained," *National Geographic* online, https://www.nationalgeographic.com/science/health-and-human-body/human-body/brain/, October 15, 2009.

5. Bruce Fischl and Anders M. Dale, "Measuring the Thickness of the Human Cerebral Cortex from Magnetic Resonance Images," *Proceedings of the National Academy of Sciences*, Vol. 97, No. 20, September 2000, 11054.

6. Editors of the Encyclopaedia Britannica, "Cerebrum," *Encyclopaedia Britannica* online, https://www.britannica.com/science/cerebrum.

7. *Ibid.*

8. Larry O. Gostin, "Ethical Considerations of Psychosurgery: The Unhappy Legacy of the Pre-frontal Lobotomy," *Journal of Medical Ethics*, Vol. 6, Iss. 3, September 1980, 149.

9. *Ibid.*

10. "Rosemary Kennedy," *John F. Kennedy Presidential Library*, https://www.jfklibrary.org/learn/about-jfk/the-kennedy-family/rosemary-kennedy.

11. Ken Kesey, *One Flew Over the Cuckoo's Nest* (New York: Viking Press, 1962); film directed by Milos Forman, starring Jack Nicholson, Louise Fletcher, 1975.

12. "Temporal Lobe Seizures," *Cleveland Clinic*, https://my.clevelandclinic.org/health/diseases/17778-temporal-lobe-seizures.

13. "What Is Epilepsy?" *Epilepsy Foundation*, https://www.epilepsy.com/learn/about-epilepsy-basics/what-epilepsythe brain and epilepsy.

14. Roger S. Fisher et al., "Epileptic Seizures and Epilepsy," 471.

15. "What Happens During a Seizure," *Epilepsy Foundation*, https://www.epilepsy.com/start-here/about-epilepsy-basics/what-happens-during-seizure.

16. F.M.C. Besag, M.J. Vasey, "Prodrome in Epilepsy," *Epilepsy Behaviour,* June 2018.

17. "About Epilepsy and Seizures," *Epilepsy Society,* https://www.epilepsysociety. org.uk/facts-and-statistics#.XhJ3_C2ZMg4.

18. Thomas R. Browne and Gregory L. Holmes, *Handbook of Epilepsy* (New York: Jones & Bartlett Learning, 2008), 37.

19. FDA News Release: "FDA Approves First Drug Comprise of an Active Ingredient Derived from Marijuana to Treat Rare, Severe Forms of Epilepsy," *U.S. Food & Drug Administration,* June 25, 2018.

20. Paolo Tinuper, Angelina Cerullo, Carla Marini, Patrizia Avoni, Anna Rosati, Roberto Riva, Agostino Baruzzi and Elio Lugaresi, "Epileptic Drop Attacks in Partial Epilepsy: Clinical Features, Evolution, and Prognosis," *Journal of Neurology, Neurosurgery & Psychiatry,* Vol. 64, Iss. 2, February 1, 1998, 231.

21. *Ibid.,* 236.

22. "Epilepsy Data and Statistics," *Centers for Disease Control and Prevention,* https://www.cdc.gov/epilepsy/data/index.html.

Chapter 4

1. J.R. Kirkup, "The History and Evolution of Surgical Instruments," *Annals of the Royal College of Surgeons of England,* Vol. 63, 1981, 279.

2. See Gary Hunter, Lady Diana Ladino, José Fransisco Tellez-Zenteno, "Art and Epilepsy Surgery," *Epilepsy & Behavior,* August 2013.

3. Owsei Temkin, *The Falling Sickness: A History of Epilepsy from the Greeks to the Beginnings of Modern Neurology* (Baltimore: Johns Hopkins University Press), 1971, 3–4.

4. Edward H. Reynolds and James V. Kinnier, "Psychoses of Epilepsy in Babylon: The Oldest Account of the Disorder," *Epilepsia,* Vol. 49, No. 9, 2008, 1490.

5. Joseph W. Schneider and Peter Conrad, "The Historical and Social Realities of Epilepsy," in *Having Epilepsy* (Philadelphia: Temple University Press, 2009), 24.

6. Sissela Bok, "The Limits of Confidentiality," *The Hastings Center Report,* Vol. 13, No. 1, February 1983, 29–30.

7. *Ibid.,* 30.

8. Richard Light, "A Real Horror Story: The Abuse of Disabled People's Human Rights," *Disability World* webzine issue number 18, April-May, 2003.

9. Tahir Obeid et al., "Possession by 'Jinn' as a Cause of Epilepsy (Saraa): A Study from Saudi Arabia," *Seizure,* Vol. 21, Iss. 4, May 2012.

10. "The History and Stigma of Epilepsy," *Epilepsia,* Vol. 4, Supp. 6, 2003, 12.

11. Marten Stol, *Epilepsy in Babylonia* (Leiden: Brill, 1993), 143.

12. Jane McCagh, "Epilepsy, Myths, Stereotypes & Stigma," *Brain Research Journal,* January 2010, 3–4.

13. Emmanouil Magiorkinis, Kalliopi Sidiropoulou, Aristidis Diamantis, "Hallmarks in the History of Epilepsy: Epilepsy in Antiquity," *Epilepsy & Behavior,* Vol. 17, Iss. 1, January 2010, 103.

14. J. V. Kinnier and E. H. Reynolds, "Text and Documents: Translation and Analysis of a Cuneiform Text Forming Part of a Treatise on Epilepsy," *Medical History,* Vol. 34, No. 2, April 1990.

15. *Ibid.,* 187.

16. *Ibid.,* 193.

17. *Ibid.,* 189.

18. Magiorkinis et al., "Hallmarks in the History of Epilepsy: Epilepsy in Antiquity," 104.

19. Joe Hitchcock, "The History of Epilepsy: An Interactive Timeline," *OUP Blog,* https://blog.oup.com/2015/03/purple-day-history-epilepsy-timeline/, March 25, 2015.

20. See Edward H. Reynolds and Michael R. Trimble, "History of Epilepsy 1909–2009: The ILAE Century," *Epilepsia,* Vol 50, Sup. 3, March, 2009.

21. Sarah Francis, "'Under the Influence'—The Physiology and Therapeutics of 'Akrasia' in Aristotle's Ethics," *The Classical Association,* Vol. 51, No. 1, May 2011, n. 212.

22. Rosemarie Kobau, Frank Gillam, David J. Thurman, "Prevalence of Self-Reported Epilepsy or Seizure Disorder and Its Associations with Self-Reported Depression and Anxiety: Results from the 2004 HealthStyles Survey," *Epilepsia,* Vol. 11, November 2006.

23. Sarah Francis, "'Under the Influence,'" 153.

24. For an in depth discussion see Owsei Temkin, *The Falling Sickness,* 148–161.

25. See Orrin Devinsky and George Lai, rev, "Spirituality and Religion in Epilepsy," *Epilepsy& Behavior,* Vol. 12, 2008.

26. Hippocrates, *On the Sacred Disease,* trans. by Francis Adams, *The Internet Classics Archive,* http://classics.mit.edu/Hippocrates/sacred.html.

27. Magiorkinis et al., "Hallmarks in the History of Epilepsy: Epilepsy in Antiquity," 104.

28. Hippocrates, *On the Sacred Disease.*

29. *Ibid.*

30. Temkin, *The Falling Sickness,* 7.

31. Hippocrates, *On the Sacred Disease.*

32. *Ibid.*

33. Susan B. Pomeroy, *Spartan Women* (New York: Oxford University Press, 2002), 34–36. Pomeroy notes that Plutarch is the only source for this, writing much later.

34. W.H.S. Jones, "Ancient Roman Folk Medicine," *Journal of Medicine and Allied Sciences,* Vol. 12, No. 4, October 1957, 465.

35. Jerome Engel, Jr., *Seizures and Epilepsy* (New York: Oxford University Press, 2012), 35.

36. "Hallmarks in the History of Epilepsy," 106.

37. Temkin, *The Falling Sickness,* 22–23.

38. W.H.S. Jones, "Ancient Roman Folk Medicine."

39. "Hallmarks in the History of Epilepsy," 107.

40. Pliny the Elder, *Natural History (English), Latin Texts and Translations,* http://perseus.uchicago.edu/perseus-cgi/citequery3.pl?dbname=PerseusLatinTexts&getid=1&query=Plin.%20Nat.%2028.2.

41. Richard S. McLachlan, "Julius Caesar's Late Onset Epilepsy: A Case of Historic Proportions," *The Canadian Journal of Neurological Sciences,* Vol. 37, No. 5, September 2010, 557.

42. Plutarch, *Caesar,* trans by John Dryden, *The Internet Classics Archive,* http://classics.mit.edu/Plutarch/caesar.1b.txt.

43. *Ibid.*

44. Francesco M. Gallasi and Hutan Ashrafian, "Has the Diagnosis of a Stroke Been Overlooked in the Symptoms of Julius Caesar?" *Neurological Science,* March 29, 2015.

45. Ian Sample, "Julius Caesar May Have Suffered Mini-Strokes, Doctors Say," *The Guardian,* April 14, 2015; Kristina Killgrove, "Julius Caesar's Health Debate Ignited: Stroke or Epilepsy," *Forbes,* May 15, 2001; Newser, "New Theory: Why Julius Caesar's Personality Changed," *Fox News,* https://www.foxnews.com/science/new-theory-why-julius-caesars-personality-changed, April 16, 2015.

46. *King James Bible,* Mark 9:17–20.

47. *Ibid.,* Mark 25–29.

48. "The History and Stigma of Epilepsy," *Epilepsia,* August 18, 2003.

49. Kzysztof Owczrek and Joanna Jędfzejczak, "Christianity and Epilepsy," *Polish Journal of Neurology and Neurosurgery,* Vol. 47, No. 3, 2013, 274.

50. *Ibid.*

51. "The History and Stigma of Epilepsy," 12.

52. Fr. Gabriele Amorth, *An Exorcist Tells His Story* (San Francisco: Ignatius Press, 2015).

53. Amorth, *An Exorcist Tells His Story,* Chapter "Targets of the Evil One," p. 11, e-book.

54. History.com Editors, "Inquisition," *History,* November 17, 2017, https://www.history.com/topics/religion/inquisition.

55. *"Malleus Maleficarum," Encyclopedia Britannica,* https://www.britannica.com/topic/Malleus-maleficarum.

56. Luther: "Witches should be burnt, even if they do no harm, merely for making a pact with the Devil," Lyle B. Steadman, "The Killing of Witches," *Oceania,* Vol. 56, No. 2, December 1985, 108. "John Calvin on Witchcraft," in Alan Kros, Edward Peters, eds., *Witchcraft in Europe, 400–1700: A Documentary History* (Philadelphia: University of Pennsylvania Press, 2001), 265–270.

57. Nachman Ben-Yehuda, "The European Witch Craze of the 14th to the 17th Centuries: A Sociologist's Perspective," *American Journal of Sociology,* Vol. 86, No. 1, July 1980, 1.

58. Heinrich Kramer and James Sprenger, *The Malleus Maleficarum,* reprint, trans. Montague Summers (New York: Cosimo, Inc., 2007), 136.

59. *Ibid.,* 179.

60. *Ibid.,* 134.

61. George Rosen, "Psychopathology in the Social Process: A Study of the

Persecution of Witches in Europe as a Contribution to the Understanding of Mass Delusions and Psychic Epidemics," *Journal of Health and Human Behavior*, Vol. 1, No. 3, Autumn 1960, 209.

62. Kathryn Kramer, "Shifting and Seizing: A Call to Reform Ohio's Outdated Restrictions on Drivers with Epilepsy, *Journal of Law and Health*, Vol. 22, 2009, 352, n.41.

63. Temkin, *The Falling Sickness*, 115–117.

64. Temkin, *The Falling Sickness*, 184.

65. Engel Jr., *Seizures and Epilepsy*, 387.

66. "Fits and Nervous Disorders," *Jackson's Oxford Journal* (Oxford, Eng.), September 30, 1758, 4.

67. "Foreign Intelligence: Paris," *The Pennsylvania Packet*, February 17, 1784, 2.

68. "Letter to Mayor of London," *The Times* of London, February 23, 1803, 1.

69. "The Hamburgh Mail," *The Waterford Mirror* (Waterford, Ir.) August 18, 1802, 3.

70. "A Female Philanthropist," *Lancaster Intelligencer* (Lancaster PA), February 11, 1845, 2.

71. Joseph W. Schneider and Peter Conrad, *Having Epilepsy* (Philadelphia: Temple University Press, 1983), 26–27.

72. "The Craig Colony of Epileptics," *Brooklyn Daily Eagle*, July 6, 1896, 3.

73. Simon D. Shorvon, "The Causes of Epilepsy: Changing Concepts of Etiology of Epilepsy Over the Past 150 Years," *Epilepsia*, Vol 52, No. 6, 1033.

74. David Nelson, "On the Treatment of Epilepsy," *The British Medical Journal*, Vol. 1, No. 390, June 20, 1868, 607.

75. Hitchcock, "The History of Epilepsy: An Interactive Timeline."

76. *Ibid.*

77. George K. York, III and David A. Steinberg, "Hughlings Jackson's Neurological Ideas," *Brain*, Vol. 134, Iss. 10, October 2011, 3107–3108.

78. Jerome Engel, Jr., Timothy A. Pedley, *Epilepsy: A Comprehensive Textbook* (Philadelphia: Lippincott Williams & Wilkins, 1998.

Chapter 5

1. P. Kwan and J.W. Sander, "The Natural History of Epilepsy: An Epidemiological View," *Journal of Neurology, Neurosurgery & Psychiatry*, Vol. 75, Iss. 10, October 2004, 1376.

2. Jack London, *Told in the Drooling Room* (New York: Dodd, Mead & Co., 1914).

3. *Ibid.*, 2.

4. Sally Satel, "A Better Breed of American," *New York Times*, February 26, 2006.

5. *Ibid.*

6. Trevor Burrus, "The United States Once Sterilized Thousands—Here's How the Supreme Court Allowed it," *Cato Institute*, January 27, 2016, https://www.cato.org/publications/commentary/united-states-once-sterilized-tens-thousands-heres-how-supreme-court-allowed.

7. *Ibid.*

8. Richard Lynn, *Eugenics: A Reassessment* (Santa Barbra, CA: Greenwood Publishing Group, 2001), 27.

9. Thomas C. Leonard, "Retrospectives: Eugenics and Economics in the Progressive Era," *The Journal of Economic Perspectives*, Vol. 19, No. 4, Autumn 2005, 216.

10. Garland E. Allen, "The Eugenics Record Office at Cold Spring Harbor, 1910–1940: An Essay in Institutional History," *Osiris*, 2nd Series, Vol. 2, 1986, 226.

11. Edwin Black, "Eugenics and the Nazis—the California connection," *San Francisco Chronicle*, November 9, 2003.

12. David Starr Jordan, *The Blood of the Nation: A Study of the Decay of Races Through the Survival of the Unfit* (London: American Unitarian Association, 1902).

13. *Ibid.*, 7.

14. Tony Platt, "Engaging the Past: Charles M. Goethe, American Eugenics, and Sacramento State University," *Social Justice*, Vol. 32, No. 2, 2005, states it, "to cleanse the body politic of racial and sexual impurities, resulting from the declining birthrate of the well-to-do and the 'evil of crossbreeding,'" 18–19.

15. Quoted in Charles P. Kindregan, "Sixty Years of Compulsory Eugenic Sterilization: 'Three Generations of Imbeciles' and the Constitution of the United States," *Chicago-Kent Law Review*, Vol. 43, No. 2, Fall 1966, 123.

16. *Ibid.*, 124.

17. Paul Popenoe, Roswell Hill Johnson, *Applied Eugenics* (New York: Macmillan Publishers, 1918), 184.

18. Scott Christianson, *The Last Gasp: The Rise and Fall of the American Gas Chamber* (Berkeley: University of California Press, 2010).

19. L. Pierce Clark, "A Critique of the Legal, Social and Economic Status of the Epileptic," *Journal of the American Institute of Criminal Law and Criminology*, Vol, 17, No. 2, August 1926, 218.

20. *Ibid.*, 221.

21. *Buck v. Bell*, Superintendent of State Colony Epileptics and Feeble Minded, 143 VA 310—VA Supreme Court, 1925.

22. *Buck v. Bell*, 274 U.S. 200, No. 292. Argued April 22, 1927, Decided May 2, 1927.

23. *Ibid.*, 207.

24. Philip R. Reilly, "Involuntary Sterilization in the United States: A Surgical Solution," *The Quarterly Review of Biology*, Vol. 62, No. 2, June 1987, 161.

25. Benno Müller-Hill, "The Blood from Auschwitz and the Silence of the Scholars," *History and Philosophy of the Life Sciences*, Vol. 21, No. 3, 1999, 332.

26. Glen Yeadon, *The Nazi Hydra in America: Suppressed History of a Century* (San Diego, CA: Progressive Press, 2008), 120–122.

27. Stefan Kühl, *Nazi Connection: Eugenics, American Racism, and German National Socialism* (New York: Oxford University Press, 2002), 58.

28. "Handicapped: Victims of the Nazi Era, 1933–1945," *A Teacher's Guide to the Holocaust, Holocaust Memorial*, https://fcit.usf.edu/holocaust/people/USHMMHAN.HTM.

29. Teaberry Blue, "Lj Idol Week 21: Hyperbole Is Literally Hitler," *LiveJournal*, April 6, 2010, https://teaberryblue.livejournal.com/606527.html.

30. Rosemarie Garland-Thomson, "Cultural Commentary: Transferred to an Unknown Location," *Disability Studies Quarterly*, Vol. 27, No. 4, Fall 2007.

31. *Ibid.*

32. Daniel J. Kevles, "Eugenics and Human Rights," *British Medical Journal*, Vol. 319, August 14, 1999, 438.

33. "Medicine, Rights for Epileptics," *Time*, December 20, 1954.

34. World Health Organization, "Epilepsy: The Public Health Aspects," *Atlas:*

Epilepsy Care in the World (Geneva: WHO, 2005), 72.

35. Lex Frieden, "Goodman and United States V. Georgia: The Supreme Court Hears Another Case Challenging the Constitutionality of Title II of the Americans with Disabilities Act," *National Council on Disability*, November 8, 2005, https://ncd.gov/publications/2005/11082005.

36. Reilly, "Involuntary Sterilization in the United States," 167.

37. "Attacks on Adoption Decrees by Natural Parents to Regain Custody," *Yale Law Journal*. Vol 61, No 4, April 1952. Example, Arkansas Statutes Annotated § 56–112, 1947: "A petition to annul a final adoption decree may be filed in the court which entered the decree on any on the following grounds: (c) That the adopted person, within five years after his final adoption has developed feeble-mindedness, insanity, epilepsy, any psychosomatic or mental disturbance, venereal disease, or any incurable disease as a result of a condition existing prior to adoption unknown to the adopting parents."

Chapter 6

1. John Appleby and Jamie Dalrymple, "Cross Sectional Study of Reporting Epileptic Seizures to General Practitioners," *British Medical Journal*, Vol 320, No. 7227, January 18, 2000.

2. Nicola Swanborough, "Epilepsy Stigma Can Be Worse Than Seizures Says Psychologist," *Epilepsy Society*, https://www.epilepsysociety.org.uk/epilepsy-stigma-worse-than-seizurest-26-06-2014#.XdDlPC2ZMg4, June 26, 2014.

3. John Appleby and Jamie Dalrymple, "Cross Sectional Study."

4. Aliyah Baruchin, "Battling Epilepsy and Its Stigma," *New York Times*, February 20, 2007.

5. Erving Goffman, *Stigma: Notes on the Management of Spoiled Identity* (New York: Prentice-Hall, 1963), 1–2.

6. Heather Love, "Stigma," in Rachel Adams, Benjamin Reiss, David Serlin, Eds., *Keywords for Disability Studies* (NY City: NYU Press, 2015), 173.

7. *Ibid.*

8. Goffman, *Stigma*, 2.

9. *Ibid.*, 5.

10. Jong-Geun Seo, Jeong-Min Kim, Sung-Pa Park, "Perceived Stigma is a Critical Factor for Interictal Aggression in People with Epilepsy," *Seizure*, Vol. 30, August 2015, 106.

11. Ann Jocoby, Dee Snape, Gus A. Baker, "Epilepsy and Social Identity: The Stigma of a Chronic Neurological Disorder," *The Lancet Neurology*, Vol. 4, Iss. 3, March 2005, 173.

12. Goffman, *Stigma*, 84–85.

13. Temkin, *The Falling Sickness*, 186.

14. Goffman, *Stigma*, 31.

15. B.P. Herman, "The Evolution of Health-Quality Health Research in Epilepsy, *Quality of Life Research*, Vol. 4, No. 2, April 1995, 90.

16. From R. Ryan R, K. Kempner, A.C. Emlen, " The Stigma of Epilepsy as a Self-Concept," *Epilepsia*, Vol. 24, No. 4, August 1980.

17. "Epilepsy," World Health Organization, https://www.who.int/news-room/fact-sheets/detail/epilepsy, June 20, 2019.

18. Katie Benner, "U.S. to Resume Capital Punishment for Federal Inmates on Death Row," *New York Times*, July 25, 2019.

19. "AG Barr Orders Reinstatement of Federal Death Penalty," NBC News, https://www.nbcnews.com/politics/justice-department/ag-barr-orders-reinstatement-federal-death-penalty-n1034451, July 25, 2019.

20. See Pamela J. Thompson and Dominic Upton, "The Impact of Chronic Epilepsy on the Family," *Seizure*, Vol. 1, Iss. 1, March 1992, 43–48.

Chapter 7

1. Fred Gibson's story from interviews by Robert Dodge, Harrisonburg, VA, July 6, 2006, July 2011.

Chapter 8

1. Peggy Arazoo, interview with Robert Dodge, SILRA Home Singapore, June, 1995.

2. Sharon Lerner, "Leprosy, a Synonym for Stigma, Returns," *New York Times*, February 18, 2003, Sec F, 6.

3. "Abandoning the Stigma of Leprosy," *The Lancet*, Vol. 393, Iss. 10170, February 2, 2019, 378.

4. Ethne Barnes, *Diseases and Human Evolution* (Albuquerque, New Mexico: University of New Mexico Press, 2005), 197.

5. Frances Tan, interviewed by Robert Dodge, Singapore, November 6, 2006.

6. David Grimm, "Global Spread of Leprosy Tied to Human Migration," *Science*, Vol 308, Iss. 5724, May13, 2005, 936.

7. From Singapore *Straits Times*, as cited in A. Joshua-Raghavar, *Leprosy in Malaysia: Past, Present and Future*. Selangor, West Malaysia: Self-published and printed through donations from charitable organizations, 1991, p. 31.

8. "Editorial," *Singapore Chronicle*, July 1830, 20.

9. Over half appear in Leviticus, while others are in Deuteronomy, Kings, Chronicles, Mathew, Mark, Luke.

10. Leviticus 14:34, "When ye be come into the land of Canaan, which I give to you for a possession, and I put the plague of leprosy in a house of the land of your possession" (*King James Bible*).

11. Numbers 5:2, "Command the children of Israel, that they put out of the camp every leper, and every one that hath an issue, and whosoever is defiled by the dead" (*King James Bible*).

12. Leviticus 13:44: "He is a leprous man, he is unclean: the priest shall pronounce him utterly unclean; his plague is in his head." 45: "And the leper in whom the plague is, his clothes shall be rent, and his head bare, and he shall put a covering upon his upper lip, and shall cry, Unclean, unclean. 'and the priest shall look on him, and pronounce him unclean'" (*King James Bible*).

13. Tan Geok Kong (Dominic), interviewed by Robert Dodge, Singapore, July 29, 2005.

14. *Ibid.*

15. "Etiology of Leprosy," *New York Medical Record*, September 10, 1892, 301.

16. Francis Seow, interviewed by Robert Dodge, Singapore, June 6, 2006.

17. Tony Gould (*A Disease Apart: Leprosy in the Modern World*, New York: St. Martin's Press, 2005), 14.

18. Chia Pua Song, interviewed in Mandarin by Sabrina Chang, Singapore

American School. Singapore, September 22, 2005. Interview translated by Sabrina Chang.

19. Lim (K)AhLee, interviewed by Robert Dodge, Singapore, July23, 2005.

20. Lim Tai Cheng, interviewed in Mandarin by Chang Ya Han and responses translated by Novita Ciputra, both of Singapore American School, Singapore, October 21, 2005.

21. Geok Kong (Dominic), July 29, 2005.

22. Lee Kiat Leng, interviewed in Hokkien by JenHao Cheng of Singapore American School, translation by JenHao Cheng, April 20, 2004.

23. Singapore *Straights Times*, November 27, 2004.

24. Geok Kong (Dominic), July 29, 2005.

25. Lim (K)AhLee, July 23, 2005.

26. Goffman, *Stigma*, 106.

27. See Laura T. Coffey, "AIDS/ The Lepers of Today Have Aids," *Tampa Bay Times*, July 6, 2006, Charles Savona-Ventura, "The Modern Leper: The HIV-AIDS Victim," *Malta Times*, November 25, 2006.

Chapter 9

1. Dr. Ronald Lesser, e-mail to Robert Dodge, October 14, 2009.

2. "Bringing Epilepsy Out of the Shadows: A Global Campaign is Launched, *World Health Press Office*, Press Release WHO 48, https://www.who.int/mental_health/neurology/epilepsy/Press Release_WHO_48_1997_en.pdf?ua=1, June 19, 1997.

3. S. Jain, P.N. Tandon, "Ayurvedic Medicine and Indian Literature on Epilepsy," *Neurology Asia, Vol. 9, Supp, 1*, 57.

4. *Ibid.*

5. *Ibid.*, 58.

6. Alok Tyagi and Norman Delanty, "Herbal Remedies, Dietary Supplements, and Seizures," *Epilepsia*, Vol. 44, No. 2, 229–230, 2003.

7. *Ibid.*, 230.

8. *Ibid.*, 231–234.

9. Gerald T. Keusch, Joan Wilentz, Arthur Kleinman, "Global Health: Developing a Research Agenda," *Lancet*, February 11, 2006, Vol. 367, 525.

10. Kheng-Seang Lim, Chong-Tin Tan, "Epilepsy Stigma in Asia: The Meaning and Impact of Stigma," *Neurology Asia*, 2014; Vol. 19, No. 1, March 2014, 6.

11. *Ibid.*

12. Kheng Seang Lim, Shi Chuo Li, Josephine Casanova-Gutierrez, Chong Tin Tan, "Name of Epilepsy, Does It Matter," *Neurology Asia*, Vol. 17, No. 2, June 2012, 88.

13. *Ibid.*

14. *Ibid.* See article also for spellings in original languages.

15. Anne Underwood, Jerry Adler, Eric Paper, "When Cultures Clash," *Newsweek International Edition*, May 16, 2005, 53.

16. Anne Fadiman, *The Spirit Catches You and You All Fall Down: A Hmong Child, Her American Doctors, and the Collision of Two Cultures* (New York: Farrar, Straus and Giroux, 1997).

17. Dr. Andrew Pan interviewed by Robert Dodge, Singapore, January 2007.

18. Eugen Trinka, Patrick Kwan, Byugin Lee, Amitabh Dash, "Epilepsy in Asia: Disease Burden, Management Barriers, and Challenges," *Epilepsia*, Vol. 6, S1, June 28, 2018, 14.

19. Lim et al., "Epilepsy Stigma in Asia," 7.

20. *Ibid.*

21. Trinka, et al., "Epilepsy in Asia," 14.

22. Kheng Seang Lim, Chin Hwan Lim, Chong Tin Tan, "Attitudes Toward Epilepsy, a Systematic Review," *Neurology Asia*, Vol. 16, No. 4, December 2011, 275.

23. Andrew Beng-Siong Pan, Shih-Hui Lim, "Public Awareness, Attitudes and Understanding Toward Epilepsy Among Singaporean Chinese," *Neurological Journal of South East Asia*, Vol. 5, June 2000, 6.

24. *Ibid.*, 10.

25. *Ibid.*, 6.

26. *Ibid.*, 9.

Chapter 10

1. Nathan B. Fountain, "Status Epilepticus: Risk Factors and Complications," *Epilepsia*, Vol. 41, Supp. 2, August 2005, S24.

2. Simon Shorvon and Monica Ferlisi, "The Outcome of Therapies in refractory and Super-Refractory Convulsive Status Epilepticus and Recommendations for Therapy," *Brain*, Vol. 135, Iss. 8, August 2012, 2319.

Chapter 11

1. See Ann Landers, "Retarded, Epileptic Sister Is Virtually Ignored by Family," *Democrat and Chronicle* (Rochester, NY) February 22, 1986, 15; "Mom Sought for Taking Retarded, Epileptic Son from Hospital," *San Francisco Examiner*, August 10, 1983, 20; united with his retarded-epileptic brother" in Sharon Cohen, "Social Services," *Los Angeles Times*, February 10, 1991, A34; "a 21-year-old retarded epileptic," in Jean Franczyk, "Deported in Error, Immokalee Woman Back from Mexico," *Miami Herald*, September 24, 1983, 189.

2. "Special Groups of Patients: Mental Retardation," *Epilepsia*, Vol. 44, Sup. 6, August 18, 2003, 79.

3. Anne T. Berg, Susan N. Smith, Daniel Frobish, Susan R. Levy, Francine M. Testa, Barbara Beckerman, Shlomo Shinnar, "Special Needs of Children with Newly Diagnosed Epilepsy," *Developmental Medicine and Child Neurology*, Vol. 47, Iss. 11, November 2005.

Chapter 12

1. *Todd's Paralysis Information Page*, https://www.ninds.nih.gov/Disorders/All-Disorders/Todds-Paralysis-Information-Page.

2. Operation description from Frederick A. Lenz, M.D., "Operative Report," *The Johns Hopkins Hospital*, Doc 39021120, May 3, 1996.

Chapter 13

1. "Neurontin (Gabapentin)," *Pfizer Medical Information*, https://www.pfizermedicalinformation.com/en-us/neurontin.

2. *Ibid.*

3. *Ibid.*

4. Hans J. Markowitsch, "Differential Contribution of Right and Left Amygdala to Affective Information Processing," *Behavioural Neurology*, Vol. 11, 1998–1999, 239.

5. *Ibid.*, 240.

6. See the following as a sample of: E.P.G. Vining, J.M. Freeman, B.S. Carson, J. Brandt, "Hemispherectomy in Children: The Hopkins Experience, 1968–1988, A Preliminary Report," *Journal of Epilepsy*, Sup. 1, 1993; Vining, E.P.G., Freeman, J.M., Pillas, D.J., Uematsu, S., Carson, B.S., Brandt, J., Boatman, D., Pulsifer, M.B., Zuckerberg, A., "Why Would You Remove Half a Brain? The Outcome of 58 Children after Hemispherectomy," *Pediatrics*, Vol. 100, 1997, 163–171; Boatman, D., Freeman, J.M. Vining, E.P.G., Pulsifer, M.B., Miglioretti, Di., Minahan, R., Carson, B.S., Brandt, J. McKhann, G., "Receptive Language after Left Hemispherectomy in Children with Late Onset Seizures, *Annals of Neurology*, Vol 46, 1999, 579–86; Kossoff, E.H., Vining, E.P.G., Pillas, D.J., Pyzik, P.L., Avellino, A.M., Carson, B.S., Freeman, J.M. Hemispherectomy for Intractable Unihemispheric Epilepsy: Etiology vs Outcome," *Neurology*, Vol. 61, 2003, 887–890; E.P.G., Vining, J.M Freeman, "Hemispherectomy—The Ultimate Focal Resection," in Luders, H., ed., *Epilepsy Surgery* (New York: Raven Press, Ltd., 1992). E.P.G. Vining, "Hemispherectomy," in O. Devinsky, Ed., *Epilepsy and Developmental Disabilities* (Charlottesville, Va: Silverchair, 2001).

7. Abigail Zuger, "Removing Half of Brain Improves Young Epileptics' Lives," *The New York Times*, Sec C, 4, August 19, 1997.

8. E.P. Vining, JM Freeman, D.J. Pillas, S. Uematsu, B.S. Carson, J. Brandt, D. Boatman, M.B. Pulsifer, A. Zuckerberg, "Why would you remove half a brain? The outcome of 58 children after hemispherectomy—the Johns Hopkins experience: 1968 to 1996," *Pediatrics*, Vol. 100, August 1997.

9. Zuger, "Removing Half of Brain Improves Young Epileptics' Lives."

10. Vining et al., "Why would you remove half a brain?"

11. Zuger, "Removing Half of Brain Improves Young Epileptics' Lives."

12. Christoph Helmstaedter, Christian Erich Elger, Juri-Alexander Witt, "The Effect of Quantitative and Qualitative Antiepileptic Drug Changes on Cognitive Recovery After Epilepsy Surgery," *Seizure*, Vol. 36, February 2016, 68.

13. C. Helmstaedter, C. E. Elger, V.L. Vogt, "Cognitive Outcomes More Than 5

Years After Temporal Lobe Epilepsy Surgery: Remarkable Functional Recovery When Seizures Are Controlled," *Seizure*, Vol. 62, https://www.sciencedirect.com/science/article/pii/S1059131118303996#!

14. *Ibid.*

15. Sonia A. Khan, "Epilepsy and Driving," *Neurosciences*, Vol. 17, No. 3, July 2017, 197.

16. See "State Driving Laws Database, *Epilepsy Foundation*, https://www.epilepsy.com/driving-laws.

17. "SMA's Letter and MOH's Reply on Doctor's Duty to Report Unfit-to-Drive Cases," *Council Notes, Singapore Medical Association*, https://www.sma.org.sg/UploadedImg/files/Publications%20-%20SMA%20News/5008/CN.pdf, November 14, 2017.

Chapter 14

1. S. Tedman, E. Thornton, G. Baker, "Development of a Scale to Measure Core Beliefs and Perceived Self Efficacy in Adults with Epilepsy." *Seizure*, Vol. 4, Iss. 3, September 1995, 228.

2. *Ibid.*

3. Marian E. Betz, Kenneth Scott, Jacqueline Jones, Carolyn DiGuiseppi, "Older Adults' Preferences for Communication with Healthcare Providers About Driving," Foundation for Traffic Safety, September 2015, 19.

4. Ronald P. Lesser, Nathan E. Crone and W.R.S. Webber, "Subdural Electrodes," Clinical Neurophysiology, Vol. 121, Iss. 9, September 2010, National Institute of Health, https://www.ncbi.nlm.nih.gov/pmc/articles/PMC2962988/#R44, June 22, 2010.

5. "Bacterial Meningitis," *Centers for Disease Control and Prevention*, https://www.cdc.gov/meningitis/bacterial.html.

6. Çagatay Önal, Hiroshi Otsub, Takashi Araki, Shiro Chitoku, Ayoko Ochi, Shelly Weiss, William Logan, Irene Elliot, O. Carter Snead III, and James T. Rutka, "Complications of Invasive Subdural Grid Monitoring in Children with Epilepsy," *Journal of Neurosurgery*, Vol. 98, May 2003, 1020–1023.

7. Jorge G. Burneo, David A. Steven, Richard S. McLachlan and Andrew G. Parrent, " Morbidity Associated with the

Use of Intracranial Electrodes for Epilepsy Surgery," *Canadian Journal of Neurological Sciences*, Vol. 33, No. 2, May 2006.

8. Eleanor Coerr, *Sadako and the Thousand Paper Cranes* (New York: G.P. Putman's Sons, 1977).

9. From J.M. Harlow, "Recovery from the Passage of an Iron Bar Through the Head," Mass Med Society, Vol. 2 1868, quoted in Kieran O'Driscoll and John Paul Leach, "'No Longer Gage': An Iron Bar Through the Head, Early Observations of Personality Change After Injury to the Prefrontal Cortex," *BMJ*, December 19, 1998.

10. Kieran O'Driscoll and John Paul Leach, "'No Longer Gage': An Iron Bar Through the Head, Early Observations of Personality Change After Injury to the Prefrontal Cortex," *BMJ*, December 19, 1998.

11. John Darrell Van Horn, Andrei Irimia, Carinna M. Torgerson, Micah C. Chambers, Ron Kikinis, Arthur W. Toga, "Mapping Connectivity Damage in the Case of Phineas Gage," PLosOne, Vol. 7, No. 5, 2012.

12. "Penfield's Homunculus: A Note on Cerebral Cartography," *Journal of Neurology, Neurosurgery & Psychiatry*, Vol. 54, No. 6, April 1993, 329–330.

13. Ronald P. Lesser, Nathan E. Crone and W.R.S. Webber, "Subdural Electrodes," Clinical Neurophysiology, Vol. 121, iss. 9, September 2010, National Institute of Health, https://www.ncbi.nlm.nih.gov/pmc/articles/PMC2962988/#R44, June 22, 2010.

14. Burneo et al., "Morbidity Associated with the Use of Intracranial Elec.," 332.

Chapter 15

1. A. Parton, P. Malhotra and M. Husain, "Hemispatial Neglect," *Journal of Neurology, Neurosurgery & Psychiatry*, Vol. 75, No. 1, January 5, 2004, 16.

2. Vilayanur S. Ramachandran and Diane Rogers-Ramachandran, "Seeing the World in Half-View." *Scientific American*, https://www.scientificamerican.com/article/seeing-the-world-in-half-view/, February 1, 2009.

3. *Ibid.*

4. E. Tillerman, S. Koelsch, N. Escoffier, E. Bigand, P. Lalitte, A.D. Friedereci and D.Y. von Cramon, "Cognitive Priming in Sung and Instrumental Music: Activation of Inferior Frontal Cortex," *NeuroImage*, Vol. 31, 2006, 1778.

Chapter 16

1. "Neurontin (gabapentin): Adverse Reactions," *Pfizer Medical Information*, https://www.pfizermedicalinformation. com/en-us/neurontin/adverse-reactions.

2. "Drugs and Supplements: Lamotrigine," *Mayo Clinic*, https://www. mayoclinic.org/drugs-supplements/ lamotrigine-oral-route/proper-use/ drg-20067449.

3. "Drugs and Supplements: Gabapentin," *Mayo Clinic*, https://www. mayoclinic.org/drugs-supplements/ gabapentin-oral-route/proper-use/ drg-2006401.

4. Robert Burns, "To a Louse: On Seeing One on a Lady's Bonnet at Church," 1786, http://www.robertburns.org/ works/97.shtml.

5. "Martha Curtis' Story," *60 Minutes*, CBS Television, December 29, 1969.

6. "SUDEP Facts," *Epilepsy Foundation*, https://www.epilepsy.com/sites/ core/files/atoms/files/SUDEP%20Facts. pdf.

7. Gina Kolata, "A Risk for Sudden Death in Epilepsy That Often Goes Unmentioned," *New York Times*, August 23, 2016, D1.

8. Jennifer Couzin "When Death Strikes without Warning," *Science*, Vol. 32, July 4, No. 5885, 2008, 31.

9. Jerome Engel, Timothy A. Pedley, Jean Aicardi, *Epilepsy: A Comprehensive Textbook* (Alphen aan den Rijn, South Holland, Netherlands: Wolters Kluwer, 2008), 44.

10. Couzin "When Death Strikes," 32.

11. "Our Stories," *North American SUDEP Registry*, http://sudepregistry. org/our-stories.

12. Kolata, "A Risk for Sudden Death in Epilepsy That Often Goes Unmentioned."

13. Couzin "When Death Strikes without Warning," 32.

14. "SUDEP Facts," *Epilepsy Foundation*.

15. ·Couzin "When Death Strikes without Warning," 33.

16. *Ibid.*, 32–33.

17. Elson L. So, "What Is Known about the Mechanism Underlying SUDEP?" *Epilepsia*, Vol. 49, Sup. 9, 2008, 94.

Chapter 17

1. Earl Lane, "Each of Our Heads Inhabited by Two Persons," Longview *Daily News* (Longview, WA), October 23, 1973, 4.

2. Newsday, "2-Brain Studies Hint We're 2 Personalities," *Los Angeles Times*, November 1, 1973, 39.

3. Thomas Nage, "Brain Bisection and the Unity of Consciousness," *Synthese*, Vol. 22, No. 3/4, May 1971, 399.

4. *Ibid.*

5. Thomas Suddendorf, Jr., "What Makes Us Human," *Psychology Today* online, https://www.psychologytoday. com/us/blog/uniquely-human/201403/ what-makes-us-human, March 10, 2014.

6. Nage, "Brain Bisection," 405.

7. Jack Thomas, "Inside the Brain," *Boston Globe*, October 8, 1984, 70.

8. Helen H. Shen, "Inner Workings: Discovering the Split Mind," *Proceedings of the National Academy of Sciences of the United States of America*, Vol. 111, No. 51, December 23, 2014, 18097.

9. *Ibid.*

10. Shen, "Inner Working."

11. Benedict Carey, "Decoding the Brain's Cacophony," *New York Times*, November 1, 2011, D1.

12. Shen, "Inner Workings," Nage, "Brain Bisection," 400.

13. *Ibid.*

14. *Ibid.*

15. Nage, "Brain Bisection," 400–401.

16. Helmi L. Lutsep, C. Mark Wessinger, Michael S. Gazzaniga, *Journal of Neurology, Neurosurgery & Psychiatry*, Vol. 59, No. 54, 50.

17. Helen H. Shen, "Inner Workings."

18. Michael S. Gazzaniga, "The Split Brain Revisited," *Scientific American*, Vol. 279, No. 1, July 1998.

19. Shen, "Inner Workings."

20. Nage, "Brain Bisection," 409.

21. Joseph E. Bogen, "Further Discussion on Split-Brains and Hemispheric

Capabilities," *British Journal for the Philosophy of Science*, Vol. 28, No. 3, September 1977, 282.

22. Roger Sperry, "Consciousness, Personal Identity, and the Divided Brain," lecture, Francis Nelson Doubleday Lecture Series "The Human Mind," Smithsonian, Wash D.C., December 1977.

23. *Ibid.*, 5.

24. *Ibid.*

25. *Ibid.*, 8–9.

26. *Ibid.*, 9.

27. *Ibid.*, 10–16.

28. Thomsen, "Split Brain & Free Will," 257.

29. Joel Frohlich, "No, You're Not Left-Brained or Right-Brained," *Knowing Neurons*, https://knowingneurons. com/2018/02/15/right-left/, February 15, 2018.

30. Dietrick E. Thomsen, "Split Brain & Free Will," *Science News*, Vol. 105, No. 16, April 20, 1974, 256.

31. *Ibid.*

32. Dietrick E. Thomsen, "Split Brain & Free Will," *Science News*, Vol. 105, No. 16, April 20, 1974.

33. *Ibid.*, 27.

34. Norman J. Finkel and Steven R. Rabat, "Split-Brain Madness: An Insanity Defense Waiting to Happen," *Law and Human Behavior*, Vol. 8, No. 3/4, December 1984, 225.

35. *Ibid.*, 226.

36. *Ibid.*

37. Daniel N. Robinson, "What Sort of Persons Are Hemispheres? Another Look at 'Split-Brain' Man," *British Journal for the Philosophy of Science*, Vol. 27, No. 1, March 1976, 77.

38. Michael S. Gazzaniga, "The Split Brain Revisited," *Scientific American*, Vol. 279, No. 1, July 1998, 55.

39. Thomsen, "Split Brain," 257.

40. Gazzaniga, "The Split Brain Revisited," 51.

41. *Ibid.*, 51,53.

42. *Ibid.*, 54.

43. Sandra Blakeslee, "New Theories of Depression Focus on Brain's Two Sides," *New York Times*, January 19, 1999, F2.

44. Timothy Ferris, "Are We Free Agents, or Merely Following Our Brain's Mysterious Orders?" *The San Francisco Examiner*, February 2, 1992, 290A.

45. David J. Turk, Todd F. Heatherton, William M. Kelley, Margaret G. Funnell, Michael S. Gazzaniga and C. Neil Macrae, "Mike of Me? Self-Recognition in a Split-Brain Patient," *Nature Neuroscience*, Vol. 5, No. 9, September 2002, 841–842.

46. W.M. Kelley, J.G. Ojemann, R.D. Wetzel, C.P. Derdeydeyn, C.J. Moran, D.T. Cross, J.L. Dowling, J.W. Miller, and S.E. Petersen, "Wada Testing Reveals Frontal Lateralization for the Memorization of Words and Faces," *Journal of Cognitive Neuroscience*, Vol. 14, No. 1, January 2002.

47. Dietrick E. Thomsen, "Split Brain & Free Will," *Science News*, Vol. 105, No. 16, April 20, 1974, 256.

48. Thomas, "Inside the Brain."

49. *Ibid.*

50. Blakeslee, "New Theories of Depression Focus on Brain's Two Sides."

Chapter 18

1. Panayiotis Patrikelis, Efthymois Angelakis, Stylianos Gatonis, "Neocognitive and Behavioral Functioning in Frontal Lobe Epilepsy: A Review," *Epilepsy & Behavior*, Vol. 14, No. 1, January 1, 2009, 21–22.

Chapter 19

1. "Lamotrogine Proper Use Oral Dose—Mayo Clinic," https://www. mayoclinic.org/drugs-supplements/ lamotrigine-oral-route/proper-use/ drg-20067449?p=1, https://www. mayoclinic.org/drugs-supplements/ carbamazepine-oral-route/proper-use/ drg-20062739?p=1.

2. J. Riss, J. Cloyd, J. Gates, S. Collins, "Benzodiazepines in Epilepsy: Pharmacology and Pharmacokineticks," *Acta Neurologica Scaninivica*, Vol. 118, No. 2, August 1, 2008, 75.

3. Sheryl R. Haut, Shlomo Shinnar, Solomon L. Moshé, Christine O'Dell and Alan D. Legatt, "The Correlation Between Seizure Clustering and Convulsive Status Epilepticus in Patients with Intractable Complex Partial Seizures," *Epilepsia*, Vol. 40, No. 12, December 1999.

Chapter 20

1. "Keppra," https://www.accessdata. fda.gov/drugsatfda_docs/label/2015/021 035s093,021505s033lbl.pdf.pdf.

2. "N20135, N21505 Keppra," FDA Approved Labeling Test, March 2015, https://www.accessdata.fda.gov/drugs atfda_docs/label/2015/021035s093,02150 5s033lbl.pdf.

3. *Ibid.*

4. Fountain, "Status Epilepticus: Risk Factors."

5. Simon Shorvon and Monica Ferlisi, "The Outcome of Therapies," 2319.

6. *Ibid.*, Fig. 1.

Chapter 21

1. "Disabled," *Merriam Webster,* https://www.merriam-webster.com/dictionary/disabled.

2. "Handicapped," *Merriam Webster,* https://www.merriam-webster.com/dictionary/handicapped.

3. Sandra J. Petty, Helen Wilding, John D. Wark, "Osteoporosis Associated with Epilepsy and the Use of Anti-Epileptics—A Review," *Current Osteoporosis Reports,* February 15, 2016, https://minerva-access.unimelb.edu. au/bitstream/handle/11343/220686/ Osteoporosis%20Associated%20with%20 Epilepsy%20and%20the%20Use%20 of%20Anti-Epileptics-a%20Review. pdf?sequence=1&isAllowed=y.

4. Xavier Bohand, Laurent Simon, Eric Perrier, Hélène Mullot, Leslie Lefeuvre and Christian Plotton, "Frequency, Types, and Potential Clinical Significance of Medication-Dispensing Errors," *Clinics,* Vol. 64. No. 1, 2009, 13.

5. *Ibid.*

6. *Ibid.*, 15.

7. "Onfi Prices, Coupons and Patient Assistance Programs: Onfi Prices" *Drugs. com,* https://www.drugs.com/price-guide/ onfi.

8. "World's Most Expensive Cities Revealed," *BBC,* March 19, 2019, https:// www.bbc.com/news/business-47617-206.

9. José F. Téllez-Zenteno and Samuel Wiebe, "Long-term Outcomes Following Epilepsy Surgery: A Systematic Review and Meta-Analysis," *Brain,* Vol. 128, Iss. 5, May 2005.

10. Pamela Crawford, William W. Hall, Brian Chappell, John Collings and Avril Stewart, "Generic Prescribing for Epilepsy. Is It Safe?" *Seizure,* Vol. 5, No. 1, February 29, 1996, 5.

11. Michel J. Berg, Robert A. Gross, Lisa S. Haskins, Wendy M. Zingaro, Kenneth J. Tomaszewski d, "Generic Substitution in the Treatment of Epilepsy: Patient and Physician Perceptions," Epilepsy & Behavior, Vol. 13, Iss. 4, November 2008, 694.

12. Muhammad Atif, Muhammad Azeem and Muhammed Rehan Sarwar, "Potential Problems and Recommendations Regarding Substitution of Generic Antiepileptic Drugs: A Systematic Review of the Literature," *Sringerplus,* Vol. 5. No. 1822, February 25, 2016, 5.

13. Damien Sharkov, "NHS: Drugs Giant Pfizer Fined Record $106 M by UK," *Newsweek.com,* https://www.newsweek. com/drugs-giant-pfizer-fined-record-106-million-uk-529120, December 7, 2016.

14. Tom Espiner, "Pfizer Fined Record £84.2m for Overcharging NHS," *BBC News,* https://www.bbc.com/news/business-38233852, December 7, 2016.

Chapter 22

1. Athanasios Gaitatzis, Anthony L. Johnson, David W. Chadwick, Simon D. Shorvon and Josemir W. Sander, "Life Expectancy in People with Newly Diagnosed Epilepsy, *Brain,* Vol. 127, Iss. 11, November 2004.

2. New Jersey, California, Nevada, Delaware, Oregon, Pennsylvania.

3. "State Driving Law Database," *Epilepsy Foundation,* https://www.epilepsy. com/driving-laws/2008341/2008811.

4. Joseph F. Drazkowski, Eli S. Neiman, Joseph I. Sirven, Gary N. McAbee and Katherine H. Noe, "Frequency of Physician Counseling and Attitudes Toward Driving Motor Vehicles in People with Epilepsy: Comparing Mandatory-Reporting with a Voluntary Reporting State," *Epilepsy & Behavior,* Vol. 19, Iss. 1, September 2010. 53.

5. *Ibid.*, 54.

6. *National Lampoon: Truly Sick, Tasteless, and Twisted Cartoons.* (Chicago: Contemporary Books, 2002), 210.

7. Wanjun Cui, Rosmarie Kobau, Matthew M. Zack, Janice M. Buelow and Joan A. Austin, "Recent Changes in Attitudes of U.S. Adults Toward People with Epilepsy—Results from the 2005 *SummerStyles* and 2013 *FallStyles* Surveys, *Epilepsy & Behavior*, Vol. 52, Part A, November 2015.

8. *Ibid.*, 16.

9. Rhona Ochse, "The Relation Between Creative Genius and Psychopathology. A Historical Perspective and a New Explanation," *South African Journal of Psychology*, Vol. 21, Iss. 1, March 1, 1991, 45.

10. *Ibid.*, 50–51.

11. Tobias Dahlkvist, "The Epileptic Genius: The Use of Dostoevsky as Example in the Medical Debate over the Pathology of Genius," *Journal of the History of Ideas*, Vol. 76, No. 4, October 2015, 592.

12. *Ibid.*, 589.

13. *Ibid.*

14. John D'Ewart, "Illness and Intellect," *The British Medical Journal*, Vol. 2, No. 2707, November 17, 1912, 1423.

15. Mathew Woods, *In Spite of Epilepsy* (New York: The Cosmopolitan Press, 1913).

16. "Famous People Who Have or Had Epilepsy," *Disability World*, https://www.disabled-world.com/disability/awareness/famous/ep.php.

17. "Famous People," *German Epilepsy Museum Kork*, http://www.epilepsiemuseum.de/english/prominente.html#text2/.

18. John H. Hugh, "Did Those Famous People Really Have Epilepsy?" *Epilepsy & Behavior*, Vol. 6, Iss. 2, March 1, 2005.

19. *Ibid.*, 135–136.

20. Louwai Muhammed, "A Retrospective Diagnosis of Epilepsy in Three Historical Figures: St Paul, Joan of Arc and Socrates," *Journal of Medical Biography*, Vol. 21, Iss. 4, November 2013, 210.

21. "Number of People with Epilepsy in the United State at All-Time High, CDC Reports," *Epilepsy Foundation*, https://www.epilepsy.com/release/2017/8/number-people-epilepsy-united-states-all-time-high-cdc-reports, August 10, 2017.

22. "Prince," *Biography*, https://www.biography.com/musician/prince, October 22, 2019.

23. Kathryn Kramer, "Shifting and Seizing: A Call to Reform Ohio's Outdated Restrictions on Drivers with Epilepsy," *Journal of Health and Law*, Vol. 22, 2009, 343.

24. M.J. Jackson and D. Turkington, "Depression and Anxiety in Epilepsy, *Journal of Neurology, Neurosurgery & Psychiatry*, Vol. 76, Supp. 1, February 16, 2005, 45.

25. Marco Mula, "Depression in Epilepsy," *Current Opinion in Neurology*, Vol. 30, No. 2, April 2017, 181.

26. *Ibid.*, 183.

27. *Ibid.*, 185.

28. Paula T. Ferdandes, Dee A. Snape, Roy G. Beran and Ann Jacoby, "Epilepsy Stigma: What Do We Know and Where Next?" *Epilepsy & Behavior*, Vol. 21, Iss. 1, September 1, 2011, 59.

Sources

All references to medical records and correspondence of reports and stays at Johns Hopkins Hospital are from their medical records as delivered to the author by flash drive provided November 7, 2019.

"Abandoning the Stigma of Leprosy." *The Lancet*, Vol. 393, Iss. 10170, February 2, 2019.

"About Epilepsy and Seizures." *Epilepsy Society.* https://www.epilepsysociety.org.uk/facts-and-statistics#. XhJ3_C2ZMg4.

"AG Barr Orders Reinstatement of Federal Death Penalty." NBC News, https://www.nbcnews.com/politics/justice-department/ag-barr-orders-reinstatement-federal-death-penalty-n1034451, July 25, 2019.

Airaksinen, E.M., Matilainen, R., Mononen, T. Mustonsen, K, Partanen, J., Jokela, V., and Halogen, P. "A Population-Based Study on Epilepsy in Mentally-Retarded Children." *Epilepsia.* Vol. 41, No. 9, September 2000.

Allen, Garland E. "The Eugenics Record Office at Cold Spring Harbor, 1910–1940: An Essay in Institutional History." *Osiris*, 2nd Series, Vol. 2, 1986.

"Americans with Disabilities Act." https://legcounsel.house.gov/Comps/Americans%20With%20Disabilities%20Act%20Of %201990.pdf.

Amorth, Father Gabriele. *An Exorcist Tells His Story.* San Francisco: Ignatius Press, 2015.

"Anatomy of the Brain." *American Association of Neurological Surgeons.* https://www.aans.org/en/Patients/Neurosurgical-Conditions-and-Treatments/Anatomy-of-the-Brain.

Appleby, John, and Dalrymple, Jamie. "Cross Sectional Study of Reporting Epileptic Seizures to General Practitioners." *British Medical Journal*, Vol. 320, No. 7227, January 18, 2000.

Arazoo, Peggy. Interviewed by Robert Dodge, SILRA Home Singapore, June, 1995.

Arkansas Statutes Annotated § 56–112, 1947.

Atif, Muhammad, Azeem, Muhammad, and Rehan Sarwar, Muhammed. "Potential Problems and Recommendations Regarding Substitution of Generic Antiepileptic Drugs: A Systematic Review of the Literature." *Sringerplus*, Vol. 5. No. 1822, February 25, 2016.

"Attacks on Adoption Decrees by Natural Parents to Regain Custody." *Yale Law Journal.* Vol. 61, No. 4, April 1952.

"Bacterial Menengitis." *Centers for Disease Control and Prevention*, https://www.cdc.gov/meningitis/bacterial.html.

Barnes, Ethne. *Diseases and Human Evolution.* Albuquerque, New Mexico: University of New Mexico Press, 2005.

Baruchin, Aliyah. "Battling Epilepsy and Its Stigma." *New York Times*, February 20, 2007.

Ben-Yehuda, Nachman. "The European Witch Craze of the 14th to the 17th Centuries: A Sociologist's Perspective." *American Journal of Sociology*, Vol. 86, No. 1, July 1980.

Benner, Katie. "U.S. to Resume Capital Punishment for Federal Inmates on Death Row." *New York Times*, July 25, 2019.

Berg, Anne T., Smith, Susan N., Frobish, Daniel, Levy, Susan R., Testa, Francine M.,

Beckerman, Barbara, and Shinnar, Shlomo. "Special Needs of Children with Newly Diagnosed Epilepsy." *Developmental Medicine and Child Neurology,* Vol. 47, Iss. 11, November 2005.

Besag, F.M.C., and Vasey, M.J. "Prodrome in Epilepsy." *Epilepsy Behaviour,* June 2018.

Betz, Marian E., Scott, Kenneth, Jones, Jacqueline, and DiGuiseppi, Carolyn. "Older Adults' Preferences for Communication with Healthcare Providers About Driving." Foundation for Traffic Safety, September 2015.

Black, Edwin. "Eugenics and the Nazis—the California Connection." *San Francisco Chronicle,* November 9, 2003.

Blakeslee, Sandra. "New Theories of Depression Focus on Brain's Two Sides." *New York Times,* January 19, 1999.

Blue, Teaberry. "Lj Idol Week 21: Hyperbole Is Literally Hitler." *LiveJournal,* April 6, 2010, https://teaberryblue.livejournal.com/606527.html.

Boatman, D., Freeman, J.M. Vining, E.P.G., Pulsifer, M.B., Miglioretti, Di., Minahan, R., Carson, B.S., Brandt, J., and McKhann, G. "Receptive Language after Left Hemispherectomy in Children with Late Onset Seizures." *Annals of Neurology,* Vol. 46, 1999.

Bogen, Joseph E. "Further Discussion on Split-Brains and Hemispheric Capabilities." *British Journal for the Philosophy of Science,* Vol. 28, No. 3, September 1977.

Bohand, Xavier, Simon, Laurent, Perrier, Eric, Mullot, Heìlelne, Lefeuvre, Leslie, and Plotton, Christian. "Frequency, Types, and Potential Clinical Significance of Medication-Dispensing Errors." *Clinics,* Vol. 64. No.1, 2009.

Bok, Sissela. "The Limits of Confidentiality." *The Hastings Center Report,* Vol. 13, No. 1, February 1983.

"The Brain Is the 'Most Complex Thing in the Universe.'" *BBC* online. May 29, 2012.

"Bringing Epilepsy Out of the Shadows: A Global Campaign Is Launched." *World Health Press Office,* Press Release WHO, https://www.who.int/mental_health/neurology/epilepsy/Press Release_WHO_48_1997_en.pdf?ua=1, June 19, 1997.

Browne, Thomas R., and Holmes, Gregory L. *Handbook of Epilepsy.* New York: Jones & Bartlett Learning, 2008.

Buck v. Bell, 274 U.S. 200, May 2, 1927.

Buck v. Bell, Superintendent of State Colony Epileptics and Feeble Minded, 143 VA. 310— VA: Supreme Court, 1925.

Burneo, Jorge G., Steven, David A., McLachlan, Richard S., and Parrent, Andrew G. "Morbidity Associated with the Use of Intracranial Electrodes for Epilepsy Surgery." *Canadian Journal of Neurological Sciences,* Vol. 33, No. 2, May 2006.

Burns, Robert. "To a Louse: On Seeing One on a Lady's Bonnet at Church." 1786, http://www.robertburns.org/works/97.shtml.

Burrus, Trevor. "The United States Once Sterilized Thousands—Here's How the Supreme Court Allowed It." Cato Institute, https://www.cato.org/publications/commentary/united-states-once-sterilized-tens-thousands-heres-how-supreme-court-allowed, January 27, 2016.

Bush, George H.W. "Remarks of President George Bush at the Signing of the Americans with Disabilities Act." https://www.eeoc.gov/eeoc/history/35th/videos/ada_signing_text.html, July 26, 1990.

Carey, Benedict. "Decoding the Brain's Cacophony." *New York Times,* November 1, 2011.

Cheng, Lim Tai. Interviewed in Mandarin by Chang Ya Han, responses translated by Novita Ciputra, Singapore, October 21, 2005.

Christianson, Scott. *The Last Gasp: The Rise and Fall of the American Gas Chamber.* Berkeley: University of California Press, 2010.

Clark, L. Pierce. "A Critique of the Legal, Social and Economic Status of the Epileptic." *Journal of the American Institute of Criminal Law and Criminology,* Vol, 17, No.2, August 1926.

Coerr, Eleanor. *Sadako and the Thousand Paper Cranes.* New York: G.P. Putman's Sons, 1977.

Coffey, Laura T. "AIDS/ The Lepers of Today Have Aids." *Tampa Bay Times,* July 6, 2006.

Cohen, Sharon. "Social Services." *Los Angeles Times,* February 10, 1991.

Couzin, Jennifer. "When Death Strikes Without Warning." *Science,* Vol. 32, July 4, No. 5885, 2008.

"The Craig Colony of Epileptics." *Brooklyn Daily Eagle,* July 6, 1896.

Crawford, Pamela, Hall, William W., Chappell, Brian, Collings, John, and Stewart, Avril. "Generic Prescribing for Epilepsy. Is It Safe?" *Seizure,* Vol. 5, No. 1, February 29, 1996.

Cui, Wanjun, Kobau, Rosmarie, Zack, Matthew M., Buelow, Janice M., and Austin, Joan A. "Recent Changes in Attitudes of U.S. Adults Toward People with Epilepsy—Results from the 2005 *SummerStyles* and 2013 *FallStyles* Surveys." *Epilepsy & Behavior,* Vol. 52, Part A, November 2015.

Dahlkvist, Tobias. "The Epileptic Genius: The Use of Dostoevsky as Example in the Medical Debate over the Pathology of Genius." *Journal of the History of Ideas,* Vol. 76, No. 4, October 2015.

DeLeire, Tom. "The Wage and Employment Effects of the Americans with Disabilities Act." *Journal of Human Resources,* Vol. 35, No. 4, Autumn 2000.

Devinsky, Orrin, and Lai, George, rev. "Spirituality and Religion in Epilepsy." *Epilepsy & Behavior,* Vol. 12, 2008.

D'Ewart, John. "Illness and Intellect." *The British Medical Journal,* Vol. 2, No. 2707, November 17, 1912.

Dodge, Jane. Interviewed by Robert Dodge, Denver, Colorado, April 27, 2015.

Drazkowski, Joseph F., Neiman, Eli S., Sirven, Joseph I., McAbee, Gary N., and Noe, Katherine H. "Frequency of Physician Counseling and Attitudes Toward Driving Motor Vehicles in People with Epilepsy: Comparing a Mandatory-Reporting with a Voluntary Reporting State." *Epilepsy & Behavior,* Vol. 19, Iss. 1, September 2010.

"Drugs and Supplements: Gabapentin." *Mayo Clinic,* https://www.mayoclinic.org/drugs-supplements/gabapentin-oral-route/proper-use/drg-2006401.

"Drugs and Supplements: Lamotrigine." *Mayo Clinic,* https://www.mayoclinic.org/drugs-supplements/lamotrigine-oral-route/proper-use/drg-20067449.

"Editorial." *Singapore Chronicle,* July 1830.

Editors of the Encyclopaedia Britannica. "Cerebrum." *Encyclopaedia Britannica* online, https://www.britannica.com/science/cerebrum.

Elliot, Irene M., Lach, Lucyna, and Smith, Mary Lou. "I Just Want to Be Normal: A Qualitative Study Exploring How Children and Adolescents View the Impact of Intractable Epilepsy on Their Quality of Life." *Epilepsy & Behavior,* Vol. 7, Iss. 4, December 1, 2005.

Emlen, A.C. "The Stigma of Epilepsy as a Self-Concept." *Epilepsia,* Vol. 24, No. 4, August 1980.

Engel, Jerome, Jr. *Seizures and Epilepsy.* New York: Oxford University Press, 2012.

_____, and Pedley, Timothy A. *Epilepsy: A Comprehensive Textbook.* Philadelphia: Lippincott Williams & Wilkins, 2008.

_____, Pedley, Timothy A., and Aicardi, Jean. *Epilepsy: A Comprehensive Textbook.* Alphen aan den Rijn, South Holland, Netherlands: Wolters Kluwer, 2008.

"The Epilepsies and Seizures: Hope Through Research." *NIH.* https://www.ninds.nih.gov/Disorders/Patient-Caregiver-Education/Hope-Through-Research/Epilepsies-and-Seizures-Hope-Through, December 30, 2019.

"Epilepsy." *Mayo Clinic.* https://www.mayoclinic.org/diseases-conditions/epilepsy/symptoms-causes/syc-20350093.

"Epilepsy." *World Health Organization.* https://www.who.int/news-room/fact-sheets/detail/epilepsy, June 20, 2019.

"Epilepsy Data and Statistics." *Centers for Disease Control and Prevention.* https://www.cdc.gov/epilepsy/data/index.html.

Espiner, Tom. "Pfizer Fined Record £84.2m for Overcharging NHS." *BBC News,* https://www.bbc.com/news/business-38233852, December 7, 2016.

"Etiology of Leprosy." *New York Medical Record.* September 10, 1892.

Fadiman, Anne. *The Spirit Catches You and You All Fall Down: A Hmong Child, Her*

American Doctors, and the Collision of Two Cultures. New York: Farrar, Straus and Giroux, 1997.

"Famous People." *German Epilepsy Museum Kork,* http://www.epilepsiemuseum.de/english/prominente.html#text2/.

"Famous People Who Have or Had Epilepsy." *Disability World,* https://www.disabled-world.com/disability/awareness/famous/ep.php.

Fanulari, Melissa. "The Effects of a Disability on Labor Market Performance: The Case of Epilepsy." *Southern Economic Journal,* Vol. 58, No. 4, April 1992.

FDA News Release: "FDA Approves First Drug Comprise of an Active Ingredient Derived from Marijuana to Treat Rare, Severe Forms of Epilepsy." *U.S. Food & Drug Administration,* June 25, 2018.

"A Female Philanthropist." *Lancaster Intelligencer* [Lancaster PA], February 11, 1845.

Ferdandes, Paula T., Snape, Dee A., Beran, Roy G., and Jacoby, Ann. "Epilepsy Stigma: What Do We Know and Where Next?" *Epilepsy & Behavior,* Vol. 21, Iss. 1., September 1, 2011, 59.

Ferris, Timothy. "Are We Free Agents, or Merely Following Our Brain's Mysterious Orders?" The *San Francisco Examiner,* February 2, 1992.

Finkel, Norman J., and Rabat, Steven R. "Split-Brain Madness: An Insanity Defense Waiting to Happen." *Law and Human Behavior,* Vol. 8, No. 3/4, December 1984.

Fischl, Bruce, and Dale, Anders M. "Measuring the Thickness of the Human Cerebral Cortex from Magnetic Resonance Images." *Proceedings of the National Academy of Sciences,* Vol. 97, No.20, September 2000.

Fisher, Robert S., and Leppik, Ilo. "Debate: When Does a Seizure Imply Epilepsy?" *Epilepsia,* December 5, 2008.

_____, Robert S., Acevedo, Carlos, Arzimanoglou, Alicia, Bogacz, Cross, J. Helen, Elger, Christian E., Engel, Jerome, Jr., Forsgren, Lars, French, Jacqueline A., Glynn, Mike, Hesdorffer, Dale C., Lee, B.I., Mathern, Gary W., Moshe, Solomon L., Perucca, Emilio, Scheffer, Ingrid E. Tomson, Torbjörn, Watanabe, Masako, and Wiebe, Samuel. "ILEA Special Report: A Practical Clinical Definition of Epilepsy." *Epilepsia,* Vol. 55, No. 4, April 14, 2014.

_____, van Emde Boas, Walter, Blume, Warren, Elger, Christian, Genton, Phillip Lee, and Engel, Jerome, Jr. "Epileptic Seizures and Epilepsy: Definitions Proposed by the International League Against Epilepsy (ILAE) and the International Bureau for Epilepsy Hesdorffer (IBE)." *Epilepsia,* Vol. 6, No. 4, April 2005.

"Fits and Nervous Disorders." *Jackson's Oxford Journal.* Oxford, Eng, September 30, 1758.

"Foreign Intelligence: Paris." *The Pennsylvania Packet.* February 17, 1784.

Fountain, Nathan B. "Status Epilepticus: Risk Factors and Complications." *Epilepsia,* Vol. 41, Supp. 2, August 2005.

Francis, Sarah. "'Under the Influence'—The Physiology and Therapeutics of 'Akrasia' in Aristotle's Ethics." *The Classical Association,* Vol. 51, No. 1, May 2011.

Franczyk, Jean. "Deported in Error, Immokalee Woman Back from Mexico." *Miami Herald,* September 24, 1983.

Frieden, Lex. "Goodman and United States V. Georgia: The Supreme Court Hears Another Case Challenging the Constitutionality of Title II of the Americans with Disabilities Act." *National Council on Disability,* November 8, 2005, https://ncd.gov/publications/2005/11082005.

Frohlich, Joel. "No, You're Not Left-Brained or Right-Brained." *Knowing Neurons,* https://knowingneurons.com/2018/02/15/right-left/, February 15, 2018.

Gage, Fred H., and Muotri, Alysson R. "What Makes Each Brain Unique." *Scientific American,* March 2012.

Gaitatzis, Athanasios, Johnson, Anthony L., Chadwick, David W., Shorvon, Simon D., and Sander, Josemir W. "Life Expectancy in People with Newly Diagnosed Epilepsy." *Brain,* Vol. 127, Iss. 11, November 2004.

Gallasi, Francesco M., and Ashrafian, Hutan. "Has the Diagnosis of a Stroke Been Overlooked in the Symptoms of Julius Caesar?" *Neurological Science,* March 29, 2015.

Garland-Thomson, Rosemarie. "Cultural Commentary: Transferred to an Unknown Location." *Disability Studies Quarterly*, Vol. 27, No. 4, Fall 2007.

Gazzaniga, Michael S. "The Split Brain Revisited." *Scientific American*, Vol. 279, No.1, July 1998.

Gibson, Fred. Interviewed by Robert Dodge, Harrisonburg, VA, July 6, 2006, July 2011.

Goffman, Erving. *Stigma: Notes on the Management of Spoiled Identity.* New York: Prentice-Hall, 1963.

Gostin, Larry O. "Ethical Considerations of Psychosurgery: The Unhappy Legacy of the Pre-frontal Lobotomy." *Journal of Medical Ethics*, Vol. 6, Iss. 3, September 1980.

Gould, Tony. *A Disease Apart: Leprosy in the Modern World.* New York: St. Martin's Press, 2005.

Grimm, David. "Global Spread of Leprosy Tied to Human Migration." *Science*, Vol. 308, Iss. 5724, May 13, 2005.

"The Hamburgh Mail." *The Waterford Mirror* [Waterford, Ir.]. August 18, 1802.

"Handicapped: Victims of the Nazi Era, 1933–1945." *A Teacher's Guide to the Holocaust, Holocaust Memorial*, https://fcit.usf.edu/holocaust/people/USHMMHAN.HTM.

Harlow, J.M. "Recovery from the Passage of an Iron Bar Through the Head." Mass Med Society, Vol. 2 1868.

Haut, Sheryl R., Shinnar, Shlomo, Moshé, Solomon L., O'Dell, Christine, and Legatt, Alan D. "The Correlation Between Seizure Clustering and Convulsive Status Epilepticus in Patients with Intractable Complex Partial Seizures." *Epilepsia*, Vol. 40, No. 12, December 1999.

Helmstaedter, Christoph, Elger, C.E., and Vogt, V.L. "Cognitive Outcomes More Than 5 Years After Temporal Lobe Epilepsy Surgery: Remarkable Functional Recovery When Seizures Are Controlled." *Seizure*, Vol. 62, November 1918. https://www.sciencedirect.com/science/article/pii/S1059131118303996#!

_____, Elger, Christian Erich, and Witt, Juri-Alexander. "The Effect of Quantitative and Qualitative Antiepileptic Drug Changes on Cognitive Recovery After Epilepsy Surgery." *Seizure*, Vol. 36, February 2016.

Herman, B.P. "The Evolution of Health-Quality Health Research in Epilepsy." *Quality of Life Research.* Vol. 4, No. 2, April 1995.

Hippocrates. *On the Sacred Disease.* trans by Francis Adams, *The Internet Classics Archive*, http://classics.mit.edu/Hippocrates/sacred.html.

"The History and Stigma of Epilepsy." *Epilepsia.* Vol. 4, Sup. 6, August 18, 2003. History.com Editors.

Hitchcock, Joe. "The History of Epilepsy: An Interactive Timeline." *OUP Blog*, https://blog.oup.com/2015/03/purple-day-history-epilepsy-timeline/, March 25, 2015.

Hoffman, Mathew. "Human Anatomy." *WebMD*, http://www.webmd.com/brain/picture-of-the-brain#1.

The Holy Bible. King James version.

Hugh, John H. "Did Those Famous People Really Have Epilepsy?" *Epilepsy & Behavior*, Vol. 6, Iss. 2, March 1, 2005.

Hunter, Gary, Ladino, Lady Diana, Fransisco, and Tellez-Zenteno, José. "Art and Epilepsy Surgery." *Epilepsy & Behavior*, August 2013.

"Inquisition." *History*, https://www.history.com/topics/religion/inquisition, November 17, 2017.

Jackson, M.J., and Turkington, D. "Depression and Anxiety in Epilepsy." *Journal of Neurology, Neurosurgery & Psychiatry*, Vol. 76, supp. 1, February 16, 2005.

Jain, S., and Tandon, P.N. "Ayurvedic Medicine and Indian Literature on Epilepsy." *Neurology Asia*, Vol. 9, Sup. 1.

Jocoby, Ann, Snape, Dee, and Baker, Gus A. "Epilepsy and Social Identity: The Stigma of a Chronic Neurological Disorder." *The Lancet Neurology*, Vol. 4, Iss. 3, March 2005.

Jones, W.H.S. "Ancient Roman Folk Medicine." *Journal of Medicine and Allied Sciences*, Vol. 12, No. 4, October 1957.

Jordan, David Starr. *The Blood of the Nation: A Study of the Decay of Races Through the Survival of the Unfit.* London: American Unitarian Association, 1902.

Joshua-Raghavar, A. *Leprosy in Malaysia: Past, Present and Future.* Selangor, Malaysia: Self-published, 1991.

Kelley, W.M., Ojemann, J.G., Wetzel, R.D., Derdeydeyn, C.P., Moran, C.J., Cross, D.T., Dowling, J.L., Miller, J.W., and Petersen, S.E. "Wada Testing Reveals Frontal Lateralization for the Memorization of Words and Faces." *Journal of Cognitive Neuroscience,* Vol. 14, No. 1, January 2002.

"Keppra." *U.S. Food & Drug Administration,* https://www.accessdata.fda.gov/drugsatfda_docs/label/2015/021035s093,021505s033lbl. pdf.

Kesey, Ken. *One Flew Over the Cuckoo's Nest.* New York: Viking Press, 1962.

Keusch, Gerald T., Wilentz, Joan, and. Kleinman, Arthur. "Global Health: Developing a Research Agenda." *Lancet,* Vol. 367, February 11, 2006.

Kevles, Daniel J. "Eugenics and Human Rights." *British Medical Journal,* Vol. 319, August 14, 1999.

Khan, Sonia A. "Epilepsy and Driving." *Neurosciences,* Vol. 17, No. 3, July 2017.

Killgrove, Kristina. "Julius Caesar's Health Debate Ignited: Stroke or Epilepsy." *The Guardian,* Apr 14, 2015. Forbes, May 15, 2001.

Kim, Lois G., Johnson, Tony L., Marson, Anthony, G., and Chadwick, David W. "Prediction of Risk of Seizure Recurrance After a Single Seizure and Early Epilepsy: Further Results from the MESS Trial." *Lancet,* Vol. 5, Iss. 4, April 2006.

Kindregan, Charles P. "Sixty Years of Compulsory Eugenic Sterilization: 'Three Generations of Imbeciles' and the Constitution of the United States." *Chicago-Kent Law Review,* Vol. 43, No. 2, Fall 1966.

Kinnier, J. V., and Reynolds, E. H. "Text and Documents: Translation and Analysis of a Cuneiform Text Forming Part of a Treatise on Epilepsy." *Medical History,* Vol. 34, No. 2, April 1990.

Kirkup, J.R. "The History and Evolution of Surgical Instruments." *Annals of the Royal College of Surgeons of England,* Vol. 63, 1981.

Kobau, Rosemarie, Gillam, Frank, and Thurman, David J. "Prevalence of Self-Reported Epilepsy or Seizure Disorder and Its Associations with Self-Reported Depression and Anxiety: Results from the 2004 HealthStyles Survey." *Epilepsia,* Vol 11, November 2006.

Kolata, Gina. "A Risk for Sudden Death in Epilepsy That Often Goes Unmentioned." *New York Times,* August 23, 2016.

Kong, Tan Geok. Interviewed by Robert Dodge, Singapore, July 29, 2005.

Kossoff, E.H., Vining, E.P.G., Pillas, D.J., Pyzik, P.L., Avellino, A.M., Carson, B.S., and Freeman, J.M. "Hemispherectomy for Intractable Unihemispheric Epilepsy: Etiology vs Outcome." *Neurology,* Vol. 61, 2003.

Kramer, Heinrich, and Sprenger, James. *The Malleus Maleficarum,* reprint, trans Montague Summers. New York: Cosimo, Inc., 2007.

Kramer, Kathryn. "Shifting and Seizing: A Call to Reform Ohio's Outdated Restrictions on Drivers with Epilepsy." *Journal of Law and Health,* Vol. 22, 2009.

Kros, Alan, and Peters, Edwards, eds. *Witchcraft in Europe, 400–1700: A Documentary History.* Philadelphia: University of Pennsylvania Press, 2001.

Kühl, Stefan. *Nazi Connection: Eugenics, American Racism, and German National Socialism.* New York: Oxford University Press, 2002.

Kwan, P., and Sander, J.W. "The Natural History of Epilepsy: An Epidemiological View." *Journal of Neurology, Neurosurgery & Psychiatry,* Vol. 75, Iss. 10, October 2004.

"Lamotrogine Proper Use Oral Dose—Mayo Clinic." https://www.mayoclinic.org/drugs-supplements/lamotrigine-oral-route/proper-use/drg-20067449?p=1, https://www.mayoclinic.org/drugs-supplements/carbamazepine-oral-route/proper-use/drg-20062739?p=1.

Landers, Ann. "Retarded, Epileptic Sister Is Virtually Ignored by Family." *Democrat and Chronicle* (Rochester, NY), February 22, 1986.

Lane, Earl. "Each of Our Heads Inhabited by Two Persons." Longview *Daily News* [Longview, WA], October 23, 1973.

Lee, Lim Ah. Interviewed by Robert Dodge, Singapore, July 23, 2005.

Leng, Lee Kiat. Interviewed in Hokkien by JenHao Cheng, trans JenHao Cheng, Singapore, April 20, 2004.

Lenz, Frederick A. "Operative Report." *The Johns Hopkins Hospital*, Doc 39021120, May 3, 1996.

Leonard, Thomas C. "Retrospectives: Eugenics and Economics in the Progressive Era." *The Journal of Economic Perspectives*, Vol. 19, No. 4, Autumn 2005.

Lerner, Sharon. "Leprosy, a Synonym for Stigma, Returns." *New York Times*, February 18, 2003.

Lesser, Ronald. e-mail to Robert Dodge, October 14, 2009.

_____, Crone, Nathan E., and Webber, W.R.S. "Subdural Electrodes." *Clinical Neurophysiology*, Vol 121, Iss. 9, September 2010.

"Letter to Mayor of London." *The Times of London*. February 23, 1803.

Light, Richard. "A Real Horror Story: The Abuse of Disabled People's Human Rights." *Disability World* webzine issue number 18, April-May, 2003.

Lim, Kheng Seang, Li, Shi Chuo, Casanova-Gutierrez, Josephine, and Tan, Chong Tin. "Name of Epilepsy, Does It Matter." *Neurology Asia*, Vol. 17, No. 2, June 2012.

Lim, Kheng Seang, Lim, Chin Hwan, and Tan, Chong Tin. "Attitudes Toward Epilepsy, a Systematic Review." *Neurology Asia*, Vol. 16, No. 4, December 2011.

Lim, Kheng-Seang, and Tan, Chong-Tin. "Epilepsy Stigma in Asia: The Meaning and Impact of Stigma." *Neurology Asia*, 2014; Vol. 19, No. 1, March 2014.

London, Jack. *Told in the Drooling Room.* New York: Dodd, Mead & Co., 1914.

Love, Heather. "Stigma." In Rachel Adams, Benjamin Reiss, David Serlin, Eds., *Keywords for Disability Studies.* NY City: NYU Press, 2015.

Lutsep, Helmi L., Wessinger, C. Mark, and Gazzaniga, Michael S. *Journal of Neurology, Neurosurgery & Psychiatry* Vol. 59, No. 54.

Lynn, Richard. *Eugenics: A Reassessment.* Santa Barbra, CA: Greenwood Publishing Group, 2001.

Mackelprang, Romel W., and Salsgiver, Richard O. "People with Disabilities and Social Work: Historical and Contemporary Issues." *Social Work*, Vol. 41, No. 1, January 1996.

Magiorkinis, Emmanouil, Sidiropoulou, Kalliopi, and Diamantis, Aristidis. "Hallmarks in the History of Epilepsy: Epilepsy in Antiquity." *Epilepsy & Behavior*, Vol. 17, Iss. 1, January 2010.

"*Malleus Maleficarum.*" *Encyclopedia Britannica.* https://www.britannica.com/topic/ Malleus-maleficarum.

Markowitsch, Hans J. "Differential Contribution of Right and Left Amygdala to Affective Information Processing." *Behavioural Neurology*, Vol. 11, 1998–1999.

"Martha Curtis' Story." *60 Minutes.* CBS Television, December 29, 1969.

Mayerson, Arlen. "The History of the ADA: A Movement Perspective." *Disability Rights and Education Fund*, https://www.ohio.k12.ky.us/userfiles/1173/Classes/8431/ The%20History%20of%20the% 20ADA.pdf, 1992.

McCagh, Jane. "Epilepsy, Myths, Stereotypes & Stigma." *Brain Research Journal*, January 2010.

McLachlan, Richard S. "Julius Caesar's Late Onset Epilepsy: A Case of Historic Proportions." *The Canadian Journal of Neurological Sciences*, Vol. 37, No. 5, September 2010.

"Medicine, Rights for Epileptics." *Time* Magazine, December 20, 1954.

Merriam Webster. Online dictionary.

"Mom Sought for Taking Retarded, Epileptic Son from Hospital." *San Francisco Examiner*, August 10, 1983.

Muhammed, Louwai. "A Retrospective Diagnosis of Epilepsy in Three Historical Figures: St Paul, Joan of Arc and Socrates." *Journal of Medical Biography*, Vol. 21, Iss. 4, November 2013.

Mula, Marco. "Depression in Epilepsy." *Current Opinion in Neurology*, Vol. 30, No. 2, April 2017.

Müller-Hill, Benno. "The Blood from Auschwitz and the Silence of the Scholars." *History and Philosophy of the Life Sciences*, Vol. 21, No. 3, 1999.

Nage, Thomas. "Brain Bisection and the Unity of Consciousness." *Synthese*, Vol. 22, No. 3/4, May 1971.

National Lampoon: Truly Sick, Tasteless, and Twisted Cartoons. Chicago: Contemporary Books, 2002.

Nelson, David. "On the Treatment of Epilepsy." *The British Medical Journal*, Vol. 1, No. 390, June 20, 1868.

"Neurontin [Gabapentin]." *Pfizer Medical Information*, https://www.pfizermedical information.com/en-us/neurontin.

"Neurontin [gabapentin]: Adverse Reactions." *Pfizer Medical Information*, https://www. pfizermedicalinformation.com/en-us/neurontin/adverse-reactions.

Newsday. "2-Brain Studies Hint We're 2 Personalities." *Los Angeles Times*, November 1, 1973.

Newser. "New Theory: Why Julius Caesar's Personality Changed." *Fox News*, https:// www.foxnews.com/science/new-theory-why-julius-caesars-personality-changed, April 16, 2015.

"N20135, N21505 Keppra: FDA Approved Labeling Test, Mar 2015." *U.S. Food & Drug Administration*. https://www.accessdata.fda.gov/drugsatfda_docs/ label/2015/021035s093, 021505s033lbl.pdf.

Obeid, Tahir, Abulaban, Ahmad, Al-Ghatani, Fawazia, Rahman, Abdul, and Al-Ghamdi, Abdulaziz. "Possession by 'Jinn' as a Cause of Epilepsy (Saraa): A study from Saudi Arabia." *Seizure*, Vol. 21, Iss. 4, May 2012.

Ochse, Rhona. "The Relation Between Creative Genius and Psychopathology. A Historical Perspective and a New Explanation." *South African Journal of Psychology*, Vol. 21, Iss. 1, March 1, 1991.

O'Driscoll, Kieran, and Leach, John Paul. "'No Longer Gage': An Iron Bar Through the Head, Early Observations of Personality Change After Injury to the Prefrontal Cortex." *BMJ*, December 19, 1998.

Önal, Çagatay, Otsub, Hiroshi, Araki, Takashi, Chitoku, Ochi, Shiro Ayoko, Weiss, Shelly, Logan, William, Elliot, Irene O., Snead, Carter, III, and Rutka, James T. "Complications of Invasive Subdural Grid Monitoring in Children with Epilepsy." *Journal of Neurosurgery*, Vol. 98, May 2003.

"Onfi Prices, Coupons and Patient Assistance Programs: Onfi Prices." *Drugs.com*, https:// www.drugs.com/price-guide/onfi.

"Our Documents—Civil Rights Act 1964." *Our Documets.gov*. 1https://www.our documents.gov/doc.php?flash=true&doc=97.

"Our Stories." *North American SUDEP Registry*, http://sudepregistry.org/our-stories.

Owczrek, Kzysztof, and Jędfzejczak, Joanna. "Christianity and Epilepsy." *Polish Journal of Neurology and Neurosurgery*, Vol. 47, No. 3, 2013.

Pan, Andrew. Interviewed by Robert Dodge. Singapore, January, 2007.

_____, Beng-Siong, and Lim, Shih-Hui. "Public Awareness, Attitudes and Understanding Toward Epilepsy Among Singaporean Chinese." *Neurological Journal of South East Asia*, Vol. 5, June 2000.

Parton, A., Malhotra, P., and Husain, M. "Hemispatial Neglect." *Journal of Neurology, Neurosurgery & Psychiatry*, Vol. 75, No. 1, January 5, 2004.

Patrikelis, Panayiotis, Efthymois Angelakis, and Stylianos Gatonis. "Neocognitive and Behavioral Functioning in Frontal Lobe Epilepsy: A Review." *Epilepsy & Behavior*, Vol. 14, No. 1, January 1, 2009.

"Penfield's Homunculus: A Note on Cerebral Cartography." *Journal of Neurology, Neurosurgery & Psychiatry*, Vol. 54, No. 6, April 1993.

Petty, Sandra J., Wilding, Helen, and Wark, John D. "Osteoporosis Associated with Epilepsy and the Use of Anti-Epileptics—A Review." *Current Osteoporosis Reports*, February 15, 2016, https://minervaaccess.unimelb.edu.au/bitstream/handle/11343/220686/

Osteoporosis%20 Associated%20with%20Epilepsy%20and%20the%20Use%20of%-20Anti-Epileptics-a%20Review.pdf?sequence=1&isAllowed=y.

Phillips, Pat. "Tripartite Global Initiative on Epilepsy Announced." *Journal of the American Medical Association,* Vol. 278, Iss. 11, September 17, 1997.

Platt, Tony. "Engaging the Past: Charles M. Goethe, American Eugenics, and Sacramento State University." *Social Justice,* Vol. 32, No. 2, 2005.

Pliny the Elder. *Natural History (English), Latin Texts and Translation.* http://perseus.uchicago.edu/perseuscgi/citequery3.pl?dbname=PerseusLatinTexts&getid=1&query=Plin.%20Nat.%2028.2.

Plutarch. *Caesar.* trans by John Dryden, *The Internet Classics Archive,* http://classics.mit.edu/Plutarch/caesar.1b.txt.

Pomeroy, Susan B. *Spartan Women.* New York: Oxford University Press, 2002.

Popenoe, Paul, and Johnson, Roswell Hill. *Applied Eugenics.* New York: Macmillan Publishers, 1918.

"Prince." *Biography,* https://www.biography.com/musician/prince, October 22, 2019.

Ramachandran, Vilayanur S., and Rogers-Ramachandran, Diane. "Seeing the World in Half-View." *Scientific American,* https://www.scientificamerican.com/article/seeing-the-world-in-half-view/, February 1, 2009.

Reilly, Philip R. "Involuntary Sterilization in the United States: A Surgical Solution." *The Quarterly Review of Biology,* Vol. 62, No. 2, June 1987.

Reynolds, Edward H., and Kinnier, James V. "Psychoses of Epilepsy in Babylon: The Oldest Account of the Disorder." *Epilepsia,* Vol. 49, No. 9, 2008.

Reynolds, Edward H., and Trimble, Michael R. "History of Epilepsy 1909–2009: The ILAE Century." *Epilepsia,* Vol. 50, Sup. 3, March, 2009.

Riss, J., Cloyd, J., Gates, J., and Collins, S. "Benzodiazepines in Epilepsy: Pharmacology and Pharmacokineticks." *Acta Neurologica Scaninivica,* Vol. 118, No. 2, August 1, 2008.

Robinson, Daniel N. "What Sort of Persons Are Hemispheres? Another Look at 'Split-Brain' Man." *British Journal for the Philosophy of Science,* Vol. 27, No. 1, March 1976.

"Rosemary Kennedy." *John F. Kennedy Presidential Library.* https://www.jfklibrary.org/learn/about-jfk/the-kennedy-family/rosemary-kennedy.

Rosen, George. "Psychopathology in the Social Process: A Study of the Persecution of Witches in Europe as a Contribution to the Understanding of Mass Delusions and Psychic Epidemics." *Journal of Health and Human Behavior,* Vol. 1, No. 3, Autumn 1960.

Satel, Sally. "A Better Breed of American." *New York Times,* February 26, 2006.

Savona-Ventura, Charles. "The Modern Leper: The HIV-AIDS Victim." *Malta Times,* November 25, 2006.

Schneider, Joseph W., and Conrad, Peter. *Having Epilepsy.* Philadelphia: Temple University Press, 1983.

Schneider, Joseph W., and Conrad, Peter. "The Historical and Social Realities of Epilepsy." In Schneider, Joseph W., and Conrad, Peter. *Having Epilepsy.* Philadelphia: Temple University Press, 2009.

Seo, Jong-Geun, Kim, Jeong-Min, and Park, Sung-Pa. "Perceived Stigma Is a Critical Factor for Interictal Aggression in People with Epilepsy." *Seizure,* Vol. 30, August 2015.

Seow, Francis. Interviewed by Robert Dodge, Singapore, June 6, 2006.

Sharkov, Damien. "NHS: Drugs Giant Pfizer Fined Record $106 M by UK." *Newsweek.com,* https://www.newsweek.com/drugs-giant-pfizer-fined-record-106-million-uk-529120, December 7, 2016.

Shen, Helen H. "Inner Workings: Discovering the Split Mind." *Proceedings of the National Academy of Sciences of the United States of America,* Vol. 111, No. 51, December 23, 2014.

Shiel, William C., Jr. "Medical Definition of Epilepsy." *MedicineNet,* https://www.medicinenet.com/script/main/art.asp?articlekey=3285, December 4, 2018.

Shorvon, Simon D. "The Causes of Epilepsy: Changing Concepts of Etiology of Epilepsy Over the Past 150 Years." *Epilepsia*, Vol. 52, No. 6.

_____, and Ferlisi, Monica. "The Outcome of Therapies in Refractory and Super-Refractory Convulsive Status Epilepticus and Recommendations for Therapy." *Brain*, Vol. 135, Iss. 8, August 2012.

"SMA's Letter and MOH's Reply on Doctor's Duty to Report Unfit-to-Drive Cases." *Council Notes, Singapore Medical Association*, https://www.sma.org.sg/UploadedImg/files/Publications%20-%20SMA%20News/5008/CN.pdf, November 14, 2017.

So, Elson L. "What Is Known about the Mechanism Underlying SUDEP?" *Epilepsia*, Vol.49, Sup. 9, 2008.

Song, Chia Pua. Interviewed in Mandarin by Sabrina Chang, Singapore, September 22, 2005. Interview translated by Sabrina Chang.

"Special Groups of Patients: Mental Retardation." *Epilepsia*, Vol. 44, Sup. 6, August 18, 2003.

Sperry, Roger. "Consciousness, Personal Identity, and the Divided Brain." Lecture, Francis Nelson Doubleday Lecture Series "The Human Mind," Smithsonian, Wash D.C., December 1977.

"State Driving Law Database." *Epilepsy Foundation*, https://www.epilepsy.com/driving-laws/2008341/2008811.

Steadman, Lyle B. "The Killing of Witches." *Oceania*, Vol. 56, No. 2, December 1985.

Stocker, Pat. Interviewed by Robert Dodge, Allenspark, Colorado, September 21, 2015.

Stocker, Tom. Interviewed by Robert Dodge, Allenspark, Colorado, September 21, 2015.

Stol, Marten. *Epilepsy in Babylonia*. Leiden: Brill, 1993.

Straits Times [Singapore], November 27, 2004.

Suddendorf, Thomas, Jr. "What Makes Us Human." *Psychology Today* online, https://www.psychologytoday.com/us/blog/uniquely-human/201403/what-makes-us-human, March 10, 2014.

"SUDEP Facts." *Epilepsy Foundation*, https://www.epilepsy.com/sites/core/files/atoms/files/SUDEP%20Facts.pdf.

Swanborough, Nicola. "Epilepsy Stigma Can Be Worse Than Seizures Says Psychologist." *Epilepsy Society*, https://www.epilepsysociety.org.uk/epilepsy-stigma-worse-than-seizurest-26–06–2014#.XdDlPC2ZMg4, June 26, 2014.

Tan, Frances. Interviewed by Robert Dodge, Singapore, November 6, 2006.

Tedman, S., Thornton, E., and Baker, G. "Development of a Scale to Measure Core Beliefs and Perceived Self Efficacy in Adults with Epilepsy." *Seizure*, Vol. 4, Iss. 3, September 1995.

Téllez-Zenteno, José F., and Wiebe, Samuel. "Long-term Outcomes Following Epilepsy Surgery: A Systematic Review and Meta-Analysis." *Brain*, Vol. 128, Iss. 5, May 2005.

Temkin, Owsei. *The Falling Sickness: A History of Epilepsy from the Greeks to the Beginnings of Modern Neurology*. Baltimore: Johns Hopkins University Press, 1971.

"Temporal Lobe Seizures." *Cleveland Clinic*. https://my.clevelandclinic.org/health/diseases/17778-temporal-lobe-seizures.

Thomas, Jack. "Inside the Brain." *Boston Globe*, October 8, 1984.

Thompson, Pamela J., and Upton, Dominic. "The Impact of Chronic Epilepsy on the Family." *Seizure*, Vol. 1, Iss. 1, March 1992.

Thomsen, Dietrick E. "Split Brain & Free Will." *Science News*, Vol. 105, No. 16, April 20, 1974.

Tillerman, E., Koelsch, S., Escoffier, N., Bigand, E., Lalitte, P., Friedereci, A.D., and von Cramon, D.Y. "Cognitive Priming in Sung and Instrumental Music: Activation of Inferior Frontal Cortex." *NeuroImage*, Vol. 31, 2006.

Tinuper, Paolo, Cerullo, Angelina, Marini, Carla, Avoni, Patrizia, Rosati, Anna, Roberto, Riva, Baruzzi, Agostino, and Lugaresi, Elio. "Epileptic Drop Attacks in Partial Epilepsy: Clinical Features, Evolution, and Prognosis." *Journal of Neurology, Neurosurgery & Psychiatry*, Vol. 64, Iss. 2, February 1, 1998.

Todd's Paralysis Information Page. https://www.ninds.nih.gov/Disorders/All-Disorders/Todds-Paralysis-Information-Page.

Trinka, Eugen, Kwan, Patrick, Lee, Byugin, and Dash, Amitabh. "Epilepsy in Asia: Disease Burden, Management Barriers, and Challenges." *Epilepsia*, Vol. 6, S1, June 28, 2018.

Turk, David J., Heatherton, Todd F., Kelley, William M., Funnell, Margaret G., Gazzaniga, Michael S., and Macrae, C. Neil. "Mike of Me? Self-Recognition in a Split-Brain Patient." *Nature Neuroscience*, Vol. 5, No. 9, September 2002.

Tyagi, Alok, and Delanty, Norman. "Herbal Remedies, Dietary Supplements, and Seizures." *Epilepsia*, Vol. 44, No. 2, 2003.

Underwood, Anne, Adler, Jerry, and Paper, Eric. "When Cultures Clash." *Newsweek International Edition*, May 16, 2005.

Van Horn, John Darrell, Irimia, Andrei, Torgerson, Carinna M., Chambers, Micah C., Kikinis, Ron, and Toga, Arthur W. "Mapping Connectivity Damage in the Case of Phineas Gage." PLosOne, Vol. 7, No. 5, 2012.

Vining, E.P.G. "Hemispherectomy." In Devinsky, O., Ed., *Epilepsy and Developmental Disabilities* (Charlottesville, Va: Silverchair, 2001).

_____, and Freeman, J.M. "Hemispherectomy—The Ultimate Focal Resection." In Luders, H., Ed., *Epilepsy Surgery* (New York: Raven Press, Ltd., 1992).

_____, Freeman, J.M., Carson, B.S., and. Brandt, J. "Hemispherectomy in Children: The Hopkins Experience, 1968–1988, A Preliminary Report." *Journal of Epilepsy*, Sup. 1, 1993.

_____, Freeman, J.M., Pillas, D.J., Uematsu, S., Carson, B.S., Brandt, J., Boatman, D., Pulsifer, M.B., and Zuckerberg, A. "Why Would You Remove Half a Brain? The Outcome of 58 Children after Hemispherectomy—the Johns Hopkins Experience: 1968 to 1996." *Pediatrics*, Vol. 100, Aug. 1997.

Wegner, Judith Welch. "Antodiscrimination Model Reconsidered: Ensuring Equal Opportunity Without Respect to Handicap Under Section 504 of the Rehabilitation Act of 1973." *Cornell Law Review*, Vol. 69, No. 401, 1984.

Wekerle, Hartmut. "Immune Protection of the Brain." *Journal of Infectious Diseases*, Vol. 186, Sup. 2, December 1, 2002.

"What Happens During a Seizure." *Epilepsy Foundation.* https://www.epilepsy.com/start-here/about-epilepsy-basics/what-happens-during-seizure.

"What Is Epilepsy?" *Epilepsy Foundation.* https://www.epilepsy.com/learn/about-epilepsy-basics/what-epilepsythe brain and epilepsy.

Woods, Mathew. *In Spite of Epilepsy.* New York: The Cosmopolitan Press, 1913.

World Health Organization. "Epilepsy: The Public Health Aspects." *Atlas: Epilepsy Care in the World.* Geneva: WHO, 2005.

"World's Most Expensive Cities Revealed." *BBC,* https://www.bbc.com/news/business-47617206. March 19, 2019.

Yeadon, Glen. *The Nazi Hydra in America: Suppressed History of a Century.* San Diego, CA: Progressive Press, 2008.

York, George K., III, and Steinberg, David A. "Hughlings Jackson's Neurological Ideas." *Brain*, Vol. 134, Iss. 10, Oct. 2011.

Zuckerman, Catherine. "The Human Brain Explained." *National Geographic* online, https://www.nationalgeographic.com/science/health-and-human-body/human-body/brain/, October 15, 2009.

Zuger, Abigail. "Removing Half of Brain Improves Young Epileptics' Lives." *The New York Times*, August 19, 1997.

Index

*Numbers in **bold italics** indicate pages with illustrations*